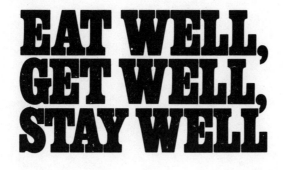

EAT WELL, GET WELL, STAY WELL

by

Carlton Fredericks, Ph.D.

GROSSET & DUNLAP
A FILMWAYS COMPANY
Publishers • New York

To two of those who have departed:
Wolfgang Seligmann, a dedicated physician
and
Bernard Workman, a friend since childhood

Contents

Introduction

Perhaps because you do not go to your physician to be kept well, the medical man is oriented toward treatment rather than prevention. Thus he is satisfied with the response in anemia to needed doses of iron, Vitamin B_6, or folic acid, even though the success of that treatment means that the disorder obviously could have been prevented with a better diet. Or he is delighted with the dramatic effect of niacinamide in returning a pellagra sufferer to sanity, although the pellagra is the product of a poor diet and could have been prevented with an adequate intake of protein and Vitamin B Complex.

Therapeutic victories in nutrition are often monuments to lost opportunities for prevention—which is to say that the kitchen may be either the escape from or the doorway to the clinic. Yet not all responses to nutritional treatment can be so characterized, for nutrients are often used to treat illnesses not caused by inadequate diet. As aspirin is not used to correct an aspirin deficiency, so Vitamin B_{12} may be employed to treat a virus disease which is obviously not caused by lack of the vitamin—shingles (herpes zoster) and cold sores (herpes simplex) being good examples. Similarly, large doses of Vitamin C may be administered to slow up the growth of a breast cancer caused by overstimulation of the breast by estrogenic (female) hormone.

1

In these therapeutic uses, the doses of nutrients needed are often very large, the healing action appearing only when the intake is far beyond that achievable through the diet. As an example, the 10 to 60 grams (1 gram = 1,000 milligrams) of Vitamin C administered daily to cancer patients, in a successful effort to extend their life expectancy, are equivalent to drinking from 100 to 600 glasses of orange juice daily. The amount of Vitamin B_6 needed to overcome excessive sensitivity to sunlight could be obtained from food by daily consumption of some 300 loaves of whole-wheat bread.

In forty years as a nutrition consultant, I have watched favorable responses—and our share of failures—in thousands of patients treated nutritionally for myriads of diseases, ranging from diabetes to hypoglycemia, from arthritis to infertility, from stammering to hyperactivity, from Raynaud's disease to Dupuytren's contracture, from atherosclerosis to arteritis to cardiac diseases, from multiple sclerosis to cerebral palsy and the epilepsies, myasthenia gravis and muscular dystrophy, from schizophrenia to depression, neurosis, and obsessive-compulsive behavior, from scleroderma to dermatomyositis, from gallbladder syndrome to gastric ulcer to regional ileitis, from senile dementia to Friedrich's ataxia—and that is a fraction of the list. Yet many physicians (and, indeed, nutritionists) as well as the public are not aware that nutrition holds benefits for patients with these and other illnesses. Hence this book: these case histories and therapies, and the lessons they teach, should obviously not be interred with me.

The histories in the book are those of real people, and their responses to nutritional treatment are real, too. In the eyes of orthodox science, these notes constitute "anecdotal evidence," which to the establishment bears the weight of patent medicine testimonials. The orthodoxy want "double-blind" studies in which one group is given a placebo, an inactive pill which appears to be the medication under test, and the other is given the active material. Neither group, nor the experimenter is aware, until the code is broken, which group is which. Often, they also want "crossover," in which the active-medication group is, without their knowledge, switched to the placebo, and vice versa. I don't worship at the shrine of the double blind, having always thought it amusingly incongruous that the scientific establishment tries so hard to rule out the healing influence of faith, but regards faith healers as ineffective quacks. More pertinent is my real apprehension that these properties of therapeutic nutrition will never be tested, or the testing delayed so long that the public will again become helpless (and suffering) victims of the cultural lag.

That my apprehension is justified, as well as what I mean by cultural lag, can be demonstrated by examining the philosophy and the statements of the Arthritis Foundation. Reflecting—and perhaps also shaping—the attitude of a majority of rheumatologists, the foundation dogmatically states that poor nutrition does not cause arthritis and that good nutrition doesn't help the arthritic. Yet the pains and impairment of joint motion in osteoarthritis—which, mitigated by aspirin, we're told we must live with—have been successfully controlled with a single vitamin. Exclusion of allergenic foods from the diet of rheumatoid arthritics has also brought significant improvement in their condition. In some cases, merely adding eggs to the diet has proved to be therapeutic. Hypertrophic arthritis has been controlled with a single vitamin and a single mineral. Cutting from the diet the nightshade plants—tomato, potato, eggplant, peppers, paprika, and tobacco—has eliminated pain and disability in thousands of patients who have a special sensitivity to a group of chemicals indigenous to these plants. A great pellagra researcher, Dr. Tom Spies, reported that he used hormones for the greater pains of arthritis but found that the lesser agonies yielded to vitamin therapy. Although this information is available in any medical library, the Arthritis Foundation still inveighs against it as "quackery," indicating that reputable practitioners will not attempt to treat arthritis nutritionally. (As you will learn later, the foundation also regarded bee venom therapy for arthritis as quackery, and made the mistake of impugning the competence of a physician who had devoted his medical life to study of this treatment; and settled the case by surrendering.)

The Arthritis Foundation is not the target of this book, but the cultural lag—widened and deepened by similar philosophies in every establishment in medicine and nutrition—is. So, if you are ill, the information here may not only help your physician to help you, but his favorable observations must induce him to pass these benefits on to other patients. As an educator I find this shortcut to medical education most appealing.

If, on the other hand, you are well, what you read here— remembering that nutrition ordinarily mitigates or prevents what it helps or cures—should inspire you to maintain good health by meeting the nutritional needs of your body and mind. Because each of us is biochemically unique, your dietary needs are likewise, demanding more careful attention to your foods and supplements if you wish to stay well, rather than lip service to "balanced meals" and the taking, when you remember it, of a multiple vitamin supplement. Further information on how to satisfy your individual nutritional needs and tolerances can be found in my book *Look Younger, Feel Healthier,* a paperback, also published by Grosset & Dunlap.

I
Notes from the
Nutritionist's Diary

I

The Making of a Nutritionist

Dr. Francis Pottenger had sent me his cat movies, showing in three generations of the animals the progress of degenerative changes we see (but count as normal because they're average) in the faces of human beings when they are products of pregnancies in which all the proteins are cooked. I decided to show the film after my evening broadcast on New York radio. It seemed unlikely that many listeners would attend at the dinner hour, and I didn't require tickets for admission. This was palpably a mistake, for we had but 500 seats, and some 4,000 people jammed the street and the lobby, with the police barring them from the elevators.

Mrs. Fredericks, who had planned a quiet restaurant dinner for two after the event, fought her way through the crowd, telling the policeman who was blocking the way, "I'm Mrs. Fredericks." He shook his head. "You're the *fourth* Mrs. Fredericks tonight," he murmured, and *you're* not getting in, either." Betty shared the story with me over a late and unquiet dinner, for we were interrupted by a radio listener who thought she recognized me. "You *are* Carlton Fredericks, aren't you?" she asked. I pleaded guilty, and she snapped, incredulously, "*You* wear *glasses?*" I pleaded for mercy, on the grounds that my mother refused to

7

take dietary advice from me when she was pregnant. The jest turned sour decades later when the public demanded that I explain why my friend, Adelle Davis, had died—and, moreover, of cancer.

I had majored in English in my undergraduate days, not only because it's a language occasionally encountered in this country, but because I had an inchoate and tentative desire to be a writer— a journalist, perhaps, or a novelist. That was succeeded by a decision to be a psychiatrist, which vanished when I took my B.A. degree into the job market of the Great Depression. Though I had but a year of chemistry, I wound up as an assistant chemist in a germicide company, a fact known to thousands of curious readers and students who have asked me how I happened to find myself in the field of nutrition. Since then I have been involved for forty years in a continuous and virulent battle with government agencies, with medical, dental, and psychiatric societies, with the nutrition departments of giant universities, with the food-processing industry and its trade associations, and with the establishments in dietetics, nutrition, cancer, arthritis, cerebral palsy, multiple sclerosis, and myasthenia gravis, not to mention vegetarians, fruitarians, fluoridationists, water distillers, the Better Business Bureaus, and several writers who have eked out a precarious, lifetime living by maligning me. At one point, my morning greeting to Betty became: "Who's attacking this morning?" And she invariably replied, "When they stop, start worrying—it will mean they think you're losing your effectiveness." During the storm of abuse, many readers, listeners, and university students asked me how I managed to continue teaching, broadcasting, lecturing, and writing. In part, my obviously irrational tenacity sprang from my certainty that the American diet was— and still is—a disaster responsible for much of our physical and mental illnesses. In part it came from a clear perspective on the dividends obtained from corrected nutrition. An even stronger factor was the series of clinical reports from my friends in the professions—physicians, dentists, psychiatrists, osteopaths, and chiropractors—who had applied my nutritional data in the management of their patients and, sometimes, in coping with their

8

personal problems. And some of my persistence survived because one develops a protective patina when exposed for four decades to the lashing of the establishment. I must confess that in a very human way, I am sometimes irked and occasionally amused when the medical journals of today discuss as effective therapies the nutritional treatments they denominated as quackery when I first spoke of them in my broadcasts of twenty years ago.

This book will be a little autobiographical, by way of explaining in more detail how a person who is reasonably sane may be motivated into pursuing a profession which awards more bruises than bonuses. It will have a great deal to tell you about many people whose lives were changed for the better, whose sicknesses were mitigated or cured by nutrition meeting their body's requirements. Interspersed you will find some of the moments of laughter—and of tears. The laughs were not infrequent. I recall Betty asking a supermarket manager for the whereabouts of the vacuum-packed wheat germ which I had introduced to the public via radio in the 1940s, when they thought it was some kind of infection. The manager, apparently the dietetic target of a wife who tuned in on my broadcasts, snorted, "Are *you* listening to that nut, too?"

The story has a point other than the disesteem in which I was held by supermarket managers, for the mention of wheat germ brings to mind the story of a little girl for whom doses of the nutrients concentrated in that good food opened the door to normalcy. She was Bonnie, she was twelve, and she was considered at least "slow," if not retarded. Her coordination was so poor that she tripped over her own feet like a two-year-old. Bonnie came to us when Betty and I had opened a summer camp for children to demonstrate that camp menus need not be based on canned vegetables, fruits packed in heavy syrup, bologna and frankfurters seasoned with nitrites, and "bug juice"—which is camp terminology for Kool-Aid. We did serve superb nutrition. We also became experts in juvenile kleptomania, pyromania, nymphomania, satyriasis, and some others I choose to forget. And we acquired Bonnie, with her slowness and imparied coordination, because her mother, who wanted her to have the benefits of good nutrition, literally cried her into the camp, despite my uneasy feeling that in competition with her normal peers the child could not be happy. I stipulated that the pediatrician, who did prove cooperative, must authorize me to do what I could for Bonnie with nutritional therapies.

Nitrites are now being banned as carcinogenic. In our camp days, we had to have the frankfurters specially made, and they had to be smuggled in under a disguised name, because frankfurters without nitrites were then considered to be a violation of federal regulations. A government agency sternly informed me that we must call them something other than frankfurters. I suggested a label (on which they never ruled) reading: "If we had added nitrites to these, we'd have to call them frankfurters."

So Bonnie came to camp. Our campus housed whites, yellows, and blacks—200 children of every race, color, and religion and a few who seemed positively extraterrestrial—and we had no problems with the racial-religious mixture until the parents arrived on Visiting Day. For that reason, we allowed but one visit during the entire summer, which restriction carried another fringe benefit to the children: they avoided the stomachaches from the "goodies" their parents would have brought. In the eighth week of the camp season, which was not a visiting weekend, Betty called Bonnie's mother and promised a pleasant surprise if she would accept our invitation to make a trip to camp. She sat, quietly weeping, watching her "awkward," "slow" daughter dancing with precision in a chorus line and faultlessly delivering her speeches. When camp closed and school reopened, the mother called Betty and said, again in tears, "I was really afraid at camp that I was seeing what I desperately wanted to see, what I had hoped and prayed for. But Bonnie just came home from school and told me that for the first time she has been placed in a class for normal children."

Bonnie had been given a concentrate, derived from wheat germ, of nutritional factors which are removed from the vegetable oils (and bread and flour) the public buys. She also took lecithin, which I used as a source of choline and inositol to fortify further the content in these vitamins of a B Complex concentrate. These nutrients, appended to a low-carbohydrate, high-protein, moderately high fat diet, constituted Bonnie's entire nutritional program. Twelve years later, scientists at the Massachusetts Institute of Technology reported a startling breakthrough: choline was a natural stimulant to brain function, via one of the neurotransmitters. (They have yet to learn that there is a nutrient which stimulates maturation of young nerve cells and repair of damaged neurones.)

Wheat germ, a good source of all the nutrients which helped Bonnie—and many other children and adults, as you will learn—is on the market because it is removed from the white flour and bread which 94 percent of the public buy. Removed, because insects and mold are reluctant to try to live on food which has lost its nutritional integrity. So white bread and flour have a long shelf life. That explains why pragmatic nutritionists suggest that you never buy food which keeps. Buy food which spoils, and eat it before it does. And buy your grains and cereals and flour in the whole-grain form. It's better to ingest these critical nutrients in palatable food than to take them under duress because you're in trouble.

The bread industry doesn't like that kind of advice, and has long defined as "food faddism" any philosophy which doesn't embrace enriched white bread as a desirable food. The technological scheme is sound: you eat the white bread, then develop constipation, to treat which you must buy back the bran that was originally removed from the bread. That not only makes the baker and the Kellogg Company richer, it does fine things for the gastroenterologist; for if you restore the fiber to your diet too late, you develop diverticulosis, diverticulitis, hemorrhoids, polyps, or bowel cancer. The other nutrients removed from wheat flour (and from rice, barley, rye, corn, and buckwheat) and not restored in enrichment are sold for pig feed, with the result that pigs enjoy *fifteen* times the intake of vitamins and minerals specified as "adequate" for human beings. Content with these triumphs of the economics of food processing and marketing, the industry takes a dim view of nutritionists who suggest, as I have, that white bread is excellent for cleaning lampshades, wallpaper, suede shoes, and typewriter keys, and a safe way of picking up broken glass.

Over and over again, the clinical responses in many diseases to treatment with concentrated whole-grain nutrients has fascinated me. That response is illustrated in the story of Danny, who was six, retarded, and a spastic (he had cerebral palsy). Danny's physician called me from the Massachusetts Bay State Training Center, where the child was an outpatient. He had developed a deformity of his back muscles from disuse, and was being measured for a back brace. The little boy already wore two leg braces and had two crutches, and his mother, clinging to the hope that nutrition might offer some help which physiotherapy had not, had persuaded the medical man to call me. I described for him a therapy based on the neuromuscular factor from wheat-germ oil, and received the conventional, halfhearted medical assent: "It won't do any good, but it can't do any harm—go ahead."

After a month of the nutritional treatment, Danny was returned to the center for the fitting of his back brace. It didn't fit! The problem was traced to an increment of muscle tissue in the atrophied area, which the physician freely granted, nothing else having been done, had to be traced to the nutritional therapy. The doctor instructed Danny's mother to continue with it and to send us both reports monthly, which she did, embellished with snapshots of the child. In the first, Danny, on his crutches, his legs in braces, was facing the camera. In the seventh, he was riding past the camera on a two-wheeled bicycle. In the accompanying report, his mother remarked, "Danny used to be the slowest in the family, but now I have trouble keeping up with him. Last night he was drying dishes, and he laid one down too near the edge of the table. It fell, but he caught it before it hit the floor. He went down doing it, but he did do it—isn't that wonderful?" It was, for a spastic, whose muscles ordinarily don't obey his wishes. The physician told me, "It must have been that neuromuscular factor, whatever that is." P.S.: He never asked me to describe it chemically, nor did he query the laboratory which made it, which means that the patients who came after Danny were never even given a chance to participate in its benefits.

Though the existence of a neuromuscular factor in wheat-germ oil was unknown to the medical man, the fact was that the oil itself had at that time already been reported useful in the treatment of neuromuscular disorders—amyotonia congenita, for instance, a condition in small babies whose muscles are so flaccid that they can't turn their heads. To this day, a quarter of a century later, medicine still doesn't know that a long-chain waxy alcohol—present only in oil that hasn't been overprocessed, as our food oils routinely are—can be used not only to help muscle function but to stimulate repair of damaged nerves. This despite the fact that the story of Danny found its way to the medical director of a cerebral palsy group who, after seeing the pictures and history of Danny, announced that in the future nutrition would play an important role in the treatment of these unfortunate children. There's only one catch: he too never asked me about the chemical identity or the source of Danny's treatment. Nonetheless, it is the Dannys who made the long battle worthwhile. It doesn't matter if the Kellogg people call you a food faddist if you benefit a child with a nutrient removed from their cereal concoctions.

I entered the field of nutrition with the enthusiasm of the educator, little realizing the strength of the establishments in the field, nor their willingness—whenever their case was weak, which it usually was—to attack the man rather than to discuss the issue. My interest in nutrition started when I worked for the germicide company I mentioned earlier, where I had the opportunity to observe that well-fed animals showed heightened resistance to induced infections. It grew when I was on the staff of McKesson and Robbins who were then, in the early 1930s, beginning to market vitamin concentrates for injection, in the use of which it was my task to educate physicians. It burned as a bright flame when I joined a staff directed by Dr. Casimir Funk, the Polish scientist who isolated thiamin (Vitamin B_1) and originated the term *vitamin* to describe it. He used a simple term because, in 1912, he had a hunch that housewives would have to become familiar with these food chemicals! I began as a copywriter, but that assignment necessitated long hours in the library, and as my knowledge of nutrition grew, in some five years I became head of the laboratory educational staff, delivering lectures on nutrition to the professions and the public. At one of these lectures, to a group of Westchester physicians, I met a doctor who insisted that in addressing medical men, I was talking to the wrong people. "We see the public after they've made nutritional mistakes for twenty or more years—and we don't know very much nutrition, anyway," he said. "You should devote yourself to educating the public before they get into trouble." It turned out that he had a relative who was an executive at a radio station in New York, and two weeks after an audition, I found myself on the air daily with a nutrition program. I regarded it as a temporary venture, and it was—if you count some 30,000 broadcasts in forty years as a transient event.

The more I learned of nutrition, the more I wanted to know, and I applied at several universities for a curriculum in the field. In each case, I was shunted to the home economics department—obviously the only haven for a male who wanted to enter a field dominated by overweight females. That meant courses in sewing, embroidery, and household management, of which I took a jaundiced view. Of this, more later.

A source of great curiosity for my listeners and readers has been the impact of my profession on my own eating habits and those of my family. My devotees delight in the story of our young Dana, who in nursery school felt obliged to explain why he wasn't permitted to eat chocolate cake or drink soda pop. "I guess," he conjectured, "that my family is kosher." Our daughter, April, crystalized the problem of being a Fredericks child. She asked a neighbor if she had any cookies that weren't "healthy." She had never, she said, tasted that kind. My listeners, more sympathetic to my credo than to my children's problems, suggested that I print "campaign" buttons for their families as well as mine, reading: "Fredericks child—don't feed."

Today, consumer advocates appear on the scene as if by prestidigitation and earn kudos for nutritional advice I gave in my broadcasts and books of a decade ago, advice that brought down on me charges of incompetence and "food faddism," not to omit reams of unfavorable publicity from publications like *TV Guide* and *The Saturday Evening Post,* which owe much revenue to the food industry. My devoted listeners resented it, of course, although as deviants from community standards of food selection and preparation, they had their own problems. The common cause created an unusually close relationship between broadcaster and listener. I still smile gently when I remember the dear lady who wrote to the manager of Station WOR in New York, remarking, "I tuned in on Dr. Fredericks late, and he was asking us to send a dollar for something. I don't know what it was, but the dollar is enclosed, and please send whatever it is to me." And the delightful man, ninety-four years old, who responded to a commercial for a mutual fund plan and attempted to buy a ten-year contract. When the salesman gently reminded him of his age, he responded, "I think Dr. Fredericks would be hurt if I didn't have confidence in his ability to keep me going for ten more years."

Which in turn reminds me of an exchange of correspondence with a physician who was a professor emeritus at Columbia College of Physicians and Surgeons. Troubled with a painful arthritic knee, he was dosing himself with a hormone of the cortisone type when he tuned in on a broadcast in which I discussed nutritional stimulation of the body's production of that hormone. He wrote to say that the idea appealed to him for several cogent reasons: as a physician he was aware of the dangerous side reactions of such hormone treatment, and as a retired physician, it struck him that manufacturing your own cortisone internally would not only be free of danger, but very much cheaper! A few months later, he wrote to say: "Last night, as I went upstairs normally—not using just one foot to ascend each step—it struck me that if I were a religious man, I'd say 'God bless you!'—but not being one, I'll simply send my thanks."

The foregoing is prologue. In the following discussions you

15

will learn how nutritional therapies are applied to many major (and minor) disorders. We'll begin with a disturbance of body chemistry which placed one of my favorite TV hosts on a psychiatric couch when he should have been seated at a dinner table, eating a diet calculated to meet his needs.

That disorder is hypoglycemia or low blood sugar—the great imitator.

2

Letters (Some Long) from Former Hypoglycemics

I had returned to New York after taping a guest appearance on a national television program, in the course of which I discovered that my host was under psychoanalysis for "depression and a severe neurosis." The label was, of course, his psychiatrist's, who was less than pleased with me when I suggested that my friend's troubles weren't "all in his mind," weren't necessarily linked to childhood experiences in toilet training, and might be purely physical in origin.

Before the tape was aired in New York, I observed a new neighbor, whom I'd not yet met, enlisting her two small boys and three small shovels in an effort to cope with mounting snowdrifts on her driveway. I'd just cleared mine with a large tractor and snow blower, and drove over to solve her problem, which I did, welcoming her to the neighborhood and leaving without introducing myself. When her small boy later saw me on the television program, he excitedly told his mother: "Do you know who's on TV tonight? The man who cleans our driveway!"

My television friend's symptoms were easily labeled psychiatric. What other interpretation would an analyst put on an unwarranted feeling of "something terrible about to happen, but I don't know what", maniacal outbursts of rage alien to the personality and out of proportion to the stimulus, plus insomnia, difficulty in concentrating, and suicidal depression—all this in a normally happy, easygoing, tolerant, and successful person? But the same list of symptoms and some thirty-five more, including claustrophobia, impotence, frigidity, blurring of vision, blackouts, and unaccustomed stammering can be caused by low blood sugar (hypoglycemia), on which I had just written a book, after some twenty-five years of research with Herman Goodman, M.D. And so it was that I cornered my host backstage and asked him about his dietary habits, which, I knew, play an important role in creating abnormal changes in the levels of blood glucose (sugar) and in susceptible people, can trigger an endless array of physical and "mental" (or even psychotic) symptoms. When I prodded him into keeping a food diary, we discovered, to his amazement if not mine, that he was drinking about thirty cups of coffee daily, each with three teaspoons of sugar. It's easy to do when every major television production staff includes a "gopher"—a young person who must "go for" coffee and everything else.

Since excessive use of caffeine and sugar, coupled with stress, are among major contributors to low blood sugar, I suggested that my friend visit a medical nutritionist for a glucose (sugar) metabolism test. He did, and it was strongly positive, as were the results when he changed his dietary habits. On a diet as low in sugar as possible, with the carbohydrates mainly in the complex (starch) form, and adequate amounts of protein and fat, he found his symptoms slipping away until, he told me, his troubles seemed to have been nothing more than a bad dream. I could have told him that bad dreams—the kind that terrify—can also be caused by low blood sugar. They strike in the small hours of the night, when blood sugar is low in *normal* individuals, since the last meal is far behind; and in those with low blood sugar, the starved brain literally sees the whole thing as a nightmare.

There is an old English proverb which goes something like: "If every man would mend a man, then would all men be mended." It was invoked when Burt Reynolds, a friend of my television host, was forced to suspend filming a picture because he was having, he had been told, a "nervous breakdown," which refused to respond to tranquilizers, antidepressants, or psychotherapy. My TV friend, exercising his painfully gained expertise, suggested that the film star go to his doctor for a glucose tolerance test, which he did. It demonstrated that he, too, had hypoglycemia, and his "breakdown" mended itself when his dietary habits were corrected.

These histories of two nationally known figures are a fraction of the stories which have come to me from readers, students, listeners, and professionals. There is the medical man who called me to say the briefest thank-you on record: "Your book," he commented, "saved my sanity." There is the Canadian practitioner whose wife went from postpregnancy "blues" to outright psychosis—a familiar story, for pregnancy is frequently the overwhelming stress which touches off hypoglycemia in those who are both susceptible and poorly fed. He wrote to express delight in his wife's responses to the hypoglycemia diet, and added one wistful question: "Will her frigidity respond, too? She wasn't always . . . " Before I was able to reply to his letter, which took months because of the thousands I receive, he called with a brief and excited progress report: "You made her a woman again!"

Orthodox science detests "anecdotal evidence"; but an anecdote is still worth listening to as an unpublished history or an interesting story. Certainly the letters which follow deserve the attention even of those physicians hopelessly wedded to the "double-blind" philosophy. They are perfectly acceptable evidence that hypoglycemia is common, that the diagnosis is missed, and that treatment is inadequate or (for want of accurate diagnosis) misdirected. They show that a mere change in diet, with special emphasis on regular small meals, minus sugar, can rescue some patients from the psychiatric couch and the endless array of tests which, in the absence of the seldom performed glucose tolerance test, will come up with negative findings, "proving" that the patient's troubles are "all in his mind."

An electrical contractor wrote: "Although I have become—literally—a new man since finding nutrition a year ago, I thought you might like to see the enclosed glucose tolerance tests, in light of some of your recent broadcasts. Although the results are un-believable—by the way, I passed out during one of the tests—both were 'normal' according to the doctor. If you wish to use any of this information for any reason, be my guest. R.M.K."

A chiropractic orthopedist wrote: "Enclosed is a report that is considered 'normal' by the local hospital. The fourth and fifth hours appear abnormal to me, based on my interpretation of your findings and other sources. The patient has bouts of depression which have been relieved by a hypoglycemia diet. W.I.H., D.C."

The test graph was enclosed. It *was* abnormal. The hospital physician *did* label it as normal, relying on a widespread medical misconcept: that there is a "magic number" for blood sugar level, above which you are normal and below which you have low blood sugar. The real "magic number" is a drop in blood sugar—to whatever level—which the patient cannot tolerate. And the patient's depression, in this case, did respond when he was placed on the hypoglycemia diet—which controlled a condition the hospital called nonexistent.

A letter from an executive at one of the giant credit card companies is characteristic of thousands I've received. The letter remarked: "Seeing the recent article about you in *Cosmopolitan* magazine prompted me to write this letter, something I meant to do long ago. I would like to express my deep gratitude to you, for your nutritional advice literally saved my father's life and also benefited my own life in countless ways.

"Without going into too much detail, my father went through two years of sheer hell simply because he was suffering from undetected hypoglycemia. It wasn't until I came across your book on low blood sugar that I realized that most of his symptoms matched the ones outlined in your book. As you predicted, it was most difficult for our family to obtain a glucose tolerance test for him; our doctor, whom, incidentally, we have dropped, preferred to think of my father as a hypochondriac, alcoholic, and neurotic. Finally, my family literally demanded that the test be given. As it turned out, my father suffers from severe hypo-glycemia, but since following the diet techniques outlined in your book (and a few tips grudgingly given by the doctor), he is today a new man.

"I tremendously admire your courage in fighting all the medical and nutritional establishments in this country, and hope you continue your work for many years to come. Sincerely, L.R."

Indeed, the hypoglycemic does become a "hypochondriac," stressing symptoms considered "meaningless" because he is so devastated by so many of them that each new one becomes another straw on the unbearable load.

One of the obstacles which made low blood sugar a fighting word to orthodox physicians is the paradox that eating sugar makes the condition worse. The explanation is simple and logical: low blood sugar often results from sensitivity to dietary sugar, provoking the body into an excessive effort to oxidize (burn) it, with the result, oversimply stated, that the blood sugar drops when the patient eats sugar. But many physicians refused to surrender to the paradox, as reflected in the next letter:

"Thank you for changing my life. I am a twenty-five-year-old housewife and mother who suffered with hypoglycemia for years. I was tense, irritable, shaky, depressed, and confused. My doctor here in Atlanta had me eating a *candy bar* when I had one of my attacks. I was up to five candy bars a day.

"The moment of truth came [when] I noticed two books on my mother's coffee table. One was your *Psycho-Nutrition* and the other was your *Low Blood Sugar and You.* I thumbed through, and I recognized my symptoms—exactly! It was then that I went on a hypoglycemia diet. It took almost three months on the diet for my body to recover from the years of nutritional abuse, but then I felt like a new person! My disposition changed drastically, and physically I felt stronger than ever. I went from a size 11 to a size 6!

"My husband and my toddler are on this diet now, too. After all, it's just plain good eating. (I swear, if politicians were on it, the world would be a peaceful place.)

"Thank you for changing my life. C.D."

There are cases of low blood sugar where sweets are not the mischief-maker. Instead, it may be sensitization to almost any food, in the form of an addictive allergy; i.e., the sufferer has an irresistible craving for the very food (or foods) which may be responsible for the low blood sugar. This addiction becomes a vicious cycle, for allergy triggers hypoglycemia, and hypoglycemia can trigger allergies. In the next letter, we see a person who has no craving for sugar, so characteristic of hypoglycemics, but develops hypoglycemia anyway. She is fortunate, for her physician doesn't tell her it's "all in her mind," and has a high index of suspicion for low blood sugar. (You don't find what you're not looking for.)

She writes: "I have just finished reading your book and felt that I should inform you that there is at least one physician on the western corner of Connecticut who is aware of hypoglycemia and its treatment.

"About three years ago, I became concerned about persistent symptoms: ravenous hunger upon waking, periodic dizziness, fuzzy vision, anxiety, and impatience. I also experienced weakness and fatigue at various times during the day, especially in the later afternoon, which degenerated into a migraine headache and finally, if ignored, sleep, and which seemed to be appeased by eating. These symptoms were accompanied by an absolute hatred and intolerance of anyone who appeared before me prior to breakfast.

"I mentioned the symptoms to my gynecologist, because I feared some of them might be attributable to the contraceptive pill. When this was shown not to be responsible, my physician immediately scheduled me for a complete physical exam, including a glucose tolerance test.

"I believe mine was a four-hour test, but no matter the duration, I had to be awakened for the last blood and urine samples, and I remember being quite perturbed and possibly rude to the lab technicians who insisted on prolonging my misery. I went straight from the hospital to the nearest restaurant, and there indulged in two complete breakfasts!

"When my doctor called with the test results, he asked me how I had felt at the last withdrawal of blood for testing. I told him, and added, 'But I could have told you I'd feel that way after being up that long without eating.' I knew how I would feel but until then I had accepted other people's evaluations that it was 'all in my head.'

"The test confirmed hypoglycemia, and I was put on the high-protein, low-carbohydrate diet you recommend. Just in case it may be of interest to your studies of hypoglycemia, I will add that my body seems to be 'wise': I have never craved sweets, have always been repulsed by anything other than meat and either eggs or cheese for breakfast, and have always been attracted to meat, cheese, fruits, or nuts for snacks, and meat and vegetables for main meals.

"Thank you for your book. I now appreciate my doctor even more for having administered a test which seemed a bit senseless to me at the time. People still laugh at my ravenous appetite for breakfast, and marvel that I eat six times daily and remain 5'4" and 108 lbs., but no one laughs after I've breakfasted and I no longer feel neurotic for being hungry. C.H."

Among other interesting observations, the preceding letter brings up another facet of missed diagnosis: hypoglycemia can be the cause of a type of migraine headache. When low blood sugar appears in a person who has not abused sugar and caffeine, two possibilities deserve investigation, the first and most important being that hypoglycemia in such a person may reflect a tendency toward diabetes—as though the oversensitive pancreas, overproducing insulin in response to rises in blood sugar, eventually becomes exhausted. (That too is an oversimplification, but here I am not writing a manual for physicians.) The second possibility is that allergy to foods other than sugar may be responsible for hypoglycemia.

The stress of pregnancy appears in many letters as a prelude to low blood sugar. From a Western state came a letter with this paragraph:

"I am forty-four, mother of four children. Looking back, I think my symptoms started after the birth of my second child. By the time I was twenty-seven, I was seeking help, and was told, at that age, that I was beginning the menopause! I would just have to learn to live with it because physically I was sound as a dollar, and should live to be a hundred. So I lived with it . . . intermittently seeking help for heart disease . . . fatigue . . . dizziness . . . loss of memory, etc., etc. All

23

the time my hair was getting whiter, my body heavier, and I was able to do less each day. I kept telling myself that as long as I got the beds made in the morning, everything was not lost, but the time came when I couldn't even perform this household chore. I had been dosed with thyroid, even larger doses of hormones and tranquilizers, and nothing seemed to help. I finally asked for a blood sugar test in Great Falls because there is a lot of diabetes in the family. This was three years ago, and it has taken most of those three years to learn how to handle this dysfunction. I wouldn't know yet if it hadn't been for your article and book. . . . I feel like a twenty-year-old again—a fat twenty-year-old, maybe, but that will go in time."

The first paragraph in her letter reiterates the now familiar story, with a twist—correct diagnosis but inadequate treatment. (Which is better, at least, than the prescription of candy bars.) My correspondent began with:

"I don't know where I'd be today without the guidance in your text. I was diagnosed as a hypoglycemic about three years ago at a distant clinic. The doctor told me I'd have to be my own doctor, that diet is the answer—eat protein, don't eat sugar." With that vague directive, she remarks, "I came home, tried, failed, and became increasingly frustrated until a close friend found your article on hypoglycemia in a magazine. It's been uphill all the way since that time."

Since hypoglycemia can be a prelude to diabetes, and a genetic factor is recognized in the latter disease, it is obvious that we must consider a possible factor of heredity in low blood sugar. This occurred to the following correspondent, a Mrs. E. J.

"Our oldest son, twenty-three, just got home from four years in the navy. Two and a half years were spent overseas in Japan, and under very straining circumstances. He was overly quiet, drank too much, wouldn't talk to any of us, finally moved out and got an apartment of his own. His mind just didn't seem to function unless he'd had something to drink. . . . He didn't want to be around people, his gums were bleeding, and his teeth were just about ready to fall out. I put him on my (hypoglycemia) diet, plus lots of Vitamin C about three weeks ago. He didn't stick to it at first, but I finally took the menus right out of your book and typed them up for him . . . went grocery shopping with him and told him I didn't want to find any salad greens left in his refrigerator a week later, and I've been checking on him every day and hounding him. He's sticking to it to please me. . . . He is also starting to function again . . . to laugh, to talk, his drinking is on the wane . . . he can go out and have a good time without getting drunk. He's getting to be more like the boy who left."

The last paragraph in this letter is a logical prelude to the stories of alcoholism which follow. A brief word of explanation: all true alcoholics develop low blood sugar for two very good reasons: (1) the alcohol damages the liver, and that organ is important in regulating blood sugar; (2) the substitution of alcohol for food obviously means malnourishment, one of the precipitating factors in hypoglycemia. But there are unfortunates who develop hypoglycemia *first*, crave liquor rather than sweets, and become alcoholics *because* they are hypoglycemic. The alcoholism treatment establishment develops a selective dysperception when we talk to them about this, the response being: "We know alcoholics are hypoglycemic." That is not what we are saying, and the distinction is important, for controlling a low blood sugar which has led to alcoholism will *cure* the alcoholism. And the doughnuts, rich in sugar (five teaspoonfuls in each), and sugared coffee dispensed by all the agencies dealing with alcoholism are virtually a prescription to prolong and intensify hypoglycemia.

A letter from an alcoholic remarks: "I heard your lecture on hypoglycemia when you spoke at the International College of Applied Nutrition. Your remarks about alcoholism were brief, and to tell you the truth, I received them skeptically. I have been an alcoholic since I was sixteen years old. I have had every treatment ever mentioned in the literature, including hypnosis, psychotherapy, shock treatment, Antabuse, AA, tranquilizers— you name it, I've had it. I decided to try the hypoglycemia diet, because it seemed to me not only that my alcoholism might be caused by low blood sugar, but that I had a number of the other symptoms you mentioned as being caused by low blood sugar.

It was two months later when I suddenly stopped drinking. I took no vows, I made no promises, I simply stopped. Since then I've had an occasional drink, and for the first time in my life I've been able to stop with one or two, whereas before I always wound up in the tank at the local court or police station. God bless you!"

At one of my lectures in California, I met the man who wrote that letter. It was three years later. He was still on the wagon.

There are babies born with hypoglycemia which, if uncorrected, can threaten life itself. There are ninety-year-olds who have low blood sugar and are mistakenly labeled as senile. This letter tells the story of one such older person:

"I shall always be grateful to you for your book on low blood sugar. Seven years ago, Mother went into the hospital for surgery. Five days after she returned home, she seemed to go 'all to pieces' all at once. For seven years she suffered from many of the symptoms you describe, but worst of all were her delusions of persecution for which she held my father responsible. She is sixty-nine and he is seventy-five, as you see this didn't happen to them at a very kind age, but of course there isn't any age that it would be kind to. Three doctors suggested psychiatric care for her but not one of them suggested any tests whatsoever for chemical imbalance of any kind.

"Last August I purchased your book, and Mother was most willing to try the diet. I might add that she had been on food supplements for almost a year. In six weeks after she started the diet you outline, she seemed her normal self, and she and my father are living together again.

"I can't be sure she accepts the fact that her low blood sugar condition (at least, I must assume that was her problem, since the diet corrected it) was responsible for her strange thoughts and feelings for seven years, but just to have her be her dear self again and have both parents together is such a relief and joy for them as well as their families. For this, Dr. Fredericks, we are most grateful, and wanted you to know it. Mrs. L.R."

Some important truths emerge from what you just read. First, in this case the stress preceding the symptoms of low blood sugar was surgery. Second, when the diet relieves the symptoms, there is no need for a glucose tolerance test. A therapeutic trial which yields healing is confirmation even better than diagnostic testing. The same thinking is quite orthodox when the physician gives you cholchicine, a drug which relieves gout. If it relieves *you*, you have gout. A third point: how easy it is to diagnose an elderly woman as a senile paranoid when she is neither senile nor actually paranoid, but suffering with a physical disorder for which no tests have been performed! Last: did you note that the patient had been on vitamin supplements for a year—obviously without impact on the symptoms—before the successful diet was tried? No supplement can yield health dividends when it is an appendage to an inadequate diet. It is a supplement, not a substitute for good nutrition, not a license to eat improperly.

Some of the letters and histories are almost cryptically brief. This, for example:

"This letter is from a very grateful family in Indiana, who through the use of your book on low blood sugar ended a seventeen-year search for the answer to their son's problems. After a very rough time with both our local doctors and one of the largest hospitals in Chicago, we wound up at the New York office of a specialist in hypoglycemia whose name was supplied by your publisher. We are happy to say that our son is a *very* much changed young man. God bless you. P.H."

Searching for objective, competent diagnosis and treatment of hypoglycemia in Chicago, home of the American Medical Association, is an exercise in frustration. The AMA, in the face of the public's rising concern with low blood sugar, announced in the early 1970s that hypoglycemia is (a) a nondisease and (b) a refuge for hypochondriacs and a bonanza for unscrupulous physicians willing to exploit them. The newspapers and medical columnists, of course, quoted it all. But they had nothing to say when in 1978, at the AMA convention on the West Coast, physicians were offered a continuing education course in—you guessed it—diagnosis and treatment of hypoglycemia. One wonders why a medical society would teach physicians how to recognize and treat a "nondisease," but on that point the AMA is reticent.

From California came a comment which invokes an important

point concerning the impact of women's diets on their menstrual cycle. My correspondent wrote:

"I have used the hypoglycemia diet for only two months, but already my health has improved radically—more zest, more energy, an improved menstrual cycle. I thought I would feel deprived without jelly doughnuts and ice cream, but a steady stream of fresh fruits, vegetables, and protein seems to keep my system content.

"Because it might add to your research findings, I'd like to mention that I suffered 33 out of the 42 symptoms listed in Chapter 2 of your book, and recently paid a psychiatrist $650 to uncover why 'I wasn't getting what I wanted out of life.' Well, the problem was located in my childhood all right. In my childhood kitchen. And the solution wasn't found on the psychiatrist's couch, but on the bookshelf of my neighborhood health food store. My grandfather owned a French bakery, and my mother was a prize-winning pastry and dessert maker. Hardly a day went by in my childhood that we didn't consume some elegant (but apparently deadly) dessert. I now cook from Francyne Davis's *Low Blood Sugar Cookbook.*

"So thanks again for helping me to regain my mental and physical health. And for doing it so pleasantly. This is also the first time in my life that I've enjoyed cooking and eating. God bless you. A.H."

You can't read such letters without feeling that someone has to remind the psychiatrists and physicians that the mind-body relationship isn't a one-way street: mind affects body, but body also affects mind. But even as I write that, I remember how the distinguished psychiatrist Smith Ely Jellife was long ago laughed off the platform when he proposed the now familiar concept of psychosomatic disorders. To his insistence that the mind can make the body sick, his jeering colleagues responded by suggesting that he join the Christian Science church. There is little reason now to believe that the orthodox establishment in medicine and psychiatry will with less resistance accept the concept of the *somato*psychic, and come to grips with the realization that disturbed metabolism or improper nutrition can chemically distort thinking and twist emotions. Yet they recognize that concept explicitly when they prescribe tranquilizers and antidepressants, lithium and choline. If there were a Nobel Prize for inconsistency, the medical referees would need a King Solomon to award it.

And now we come to a gem of a first-person story from a hypoglycemic, a layman trapped in the aggravated cultural lag in medicine. This is the reasoned, passionate outcry of a college professor who escaped the psychiatric couch only because he proved—over the implacable opposition of his apathetic physicians—that he was a hypoglycemic. With him it became a crusade, exactly as I found myself, after writing a book on low blood sugar, tilting at the windmills of the medical establishment and the processed food industry. At his wish, the professor remains unidentified, as do his doctors and the hospitals which were a party to the obstructionism, our policy being to protect both the victim and the assailants.

The educator first wrote to me in April 1974. He opened with a phrase as familiar to you by now as it became to my co-author and me: "I am writing to give you my most sincere thanks for your book on low blood sugar. I believe that this book, along with my good fortune in finding it when I did, probably saved me from insanity and perhaps death.

"I had been troubled for three years by incessant fatigue, culminating in a series of morning seizures, blackouts, and episodes of dizziness and anxiety which had become progressively worse until by December of 1973 I was almost completely incapacitated. I had visited several physicians, each of whom had suggested that my problems were 'nervous reactions' and 'anxiety attacks' and had given me injections of Valium and vertigo tablets during my worst seizures. But I felt that something else was wrong since I am generally a fairly easygoing and happy person.

"My first clue that food might have something to do with my troubles came when my condition abruptly became much worse around Christmas.* On reflection I realized that the only thing

---

*Psychoanalysts will dogmatically insist that many people are depressed during holidays.

really different about Christmas was that I ate many sugar-laden foods. Although something as apparently harmless as sugar seemed an unlikely cause of such extreme troubles as I had had, I saw a copy of your book and on impulse bought it, read it, and saw that sugar could indeed cause such troubles in susceptible individuals.

"I then began following your diet, and a week later went to ———— Clinic, where I insisted on and took the glucose tolerance test. One hour after drinking the glucose (sugar) beverage I had a massive seizure that required two men to hold me in a chair, then rendered me unconscious for about twenty minutes. The lab report did not indicate hypoglycemia, perhaps because I'd been on a low carbohydrate diet for the preceding week, but the seizure indicated that sugar did indeed have an abnormal effect on me, so I was told to continue the hypoglycemia diet but was not advised to take the yeast supplement that your book recommends.

"During the following three weeks my condition improved somewhat. The stomach pains that had bothered me for years abruptly disappeared, and I had only three seizures during this period. But I began hearing a strange humming sound in my right ear, and was literally floored by severe vertigo one night late in February. I was taken to ———— Hospital, where, unsure of the tentative diagnosis of hypoglycemia, my physicians put me through ear examinations, a brain scan, EEG, cardiogram, spinal tap, neurological examinations, psychological tests, and psychiatric interviews. All results were negative, the only objectively measurable neurological symptom being that my eyes crossed. I had to wear a patch over one eye for about two weeks. My physicians, obviously unsure about hypoglycemia, prescribed psychotherapy for what some of them felt was a psychosomatic illness. I was hospitalized for ten days.

"I willingly began psychotherapy, for my anxiety, as you can imagine, had become constant and intense. But I also returned on my own to the hypoglycemia diet—this time with the yeast and glycine supplements you recommend—and now, over a month later, I am feeling better than I have in several years. I feel that the psychotherapy has not been particularly productive. My therapist usually only stares at his clock, and says, 'What does this feeling remind you of from your childhood?' And my answer is usually, 'Nothing.' But the diet and supplements seem to have worked, for I have been free of seizures, blackouts, dizziness, and most of my anxiety for about a month now. I still get tired easily, but a midday nap helps this.

"So again I thank you for your book. Being a English teacher, I am usually rather blasé about even the most sensational printed matter. But in this case one small book, discovered by accident, has made a tremendous difference, perhaps a difference between life and death. Thank you again. J.C."

He added a P.S.: "If for any reason you would like a more detailed account of my illness, I will be happy to write it for you." I invited him to do so. The result is the following saga of the layman caught in medicine's cultural lag, a victim of medicine's blind spot for nutrition. It is lengthy, but I promise that you will find it worth reading. The educator is addressing his physician at the hospital where the glucose test was pronounced "normal" although the patient had a seizure as part of his reaction to a dose of sugar, lost all his color vision, and was—unaccustomedly—stuttering. Copies of this letter went to every department of the hospital with which the clinic is affiliated, and additional copies were sent to a Senate committee which was holding hearings on a bill providing, among other considerations, encouragement for the teaching of nutrition in medical schools. The professor wrote to his physician:

"Since last I saw you two months ago my condition has continued to improve. I have remained free of most of the symptoms given you in my initial visit* six months ago, and of the vertigo and disorientation for which I was hospitalized a month later. Especially, I have had no seizures or blackouts since resuming the hypoglycemia diet with B Complex supplements after my release from the hospital, and my physical and emotional states

---

*The professor's letter contained numerous footnotes, which have been summarized in Appendix A.

have returned to nearly normal. The only symptoms I now have are occasional headaches and slight pain in my ears, occasional aches in legs and feet, frequent rectal pain and itching, occasional episodes of thirst and frequent urination, and frequent drowsiness following meals. (Food at these times does not merely make me sleepy, it puts me to sleep.)

"These symptoms seem to me patently prediabetic and, together with my relatively high blood glucose fasting level and two-hour level (104 and 120, respectively) in the glucose tolerance test, perhaps indicate that my hypoglycemia is of diabetic etiology.

"In a recent substantial study of hypoglycemia, *Personality Disorder and Reactive Hypoglycemia*, a two-hour level of 120 or greater in hypoglycemic patients is considered diabetic. I would like therefore to have sugar level tests run occasionally to keep a check on this. There is some diabetes on both sides of my family.

"To put in proper perspective what I have to say next, I would like first to say that I think you are a fine doctor. I was very grateful for the interest you took in my case before and while I was hospitalized, and I am satisfied that you did everything you knew to find out what was wrong with me and to try to correct it. You are several cuts above other doctors I have consulted over the past three years in connection with this illness, both in terms of the deliberation with which you considered my problems and the thoroughness with which you have attempted to cope with them. So I do not intend what follows as an attack upon you by any means. You and I have the same adversary in this hypoglycemia business: a grossly chaotic state-of-the-art. The research on hypoglycemia—and I know because I have been through much of it—is a confused mass of contradictions and uncertainties. But I know from firsthand experience, and hopefully you and your colleagues also know or soon will, that hypoglycemia is a real disease, an extremely serious disease, and one which demands immediate, decisive, and informed treatment.

"In spite of my respect for you, and the confusion in the scholarship, I feel that you and your colleagues, and to a much more serious extent the other physicians whom I have consulted over the past three years, have made a number of obvious and serious mistakes in your handling of my case. The principal purpose of this communication is to outline these mistakes in the hope that you can avoid making the same mistakes in the future. The fact that I have now almost completely recovered from this illness is a result not of anything that you have done or prescribed for me, but of my pursuing an intuitive awareness, resulting from my violent physical reaction to the glucose tolerance test, that sugar was in some way quite bad for me, and of my going into the library myself to try to discover just what sugar was capable of doing to the human body and psyche. What I have discovered, in essence, is that if you wait until all the clinical results are in before you begin taking hypoglycemics off sugar, you will probably have to wait for many years, by which time many hypoglycemics will be either insane or dead. There are other diseases which you do not fully understand, such as cancer and heart disease, yet you have developed certain techniques with which you attempt to cope with them. I argue that people who react violently to a dose of sugar, and in whom other diseases have been ruled out, must likewise be given the benefit of the established procedures for the treatment of reactive hypoglycemia, even if the clinical criteria for the diagnosis of this disease are not yet firmly established." [*Note:* They *are.* And have been for decades.]

"My chief concern is not for myself, but for other hypoglycemics who might come to the ———— Clinic and be handled in the way I was handled. I never again want a reactive hypoglycemic in such bad shape as I was to be put through the tortures I endured in the hospital and then to be thrown into the catchall bag of psychosomatic medicine, from which, for the undiagnosed hypoglycemic, there is often no escape. This illness itself is horrible beyond all description, and for physicians to make it worse instead of better borders on the kind of misconduct more characteristic of Buchenwald and Dachau than ———— Hospital.

"Your first mistake was in essentially ignoring my observation that sugar seemed to make my condition worse. If a patient comes to you saying that he has a pain in his stomach, do you insist that the pain is really in his toes instead? I tend to believe that a patient's own subjective judgments about his condition can often be quite helpful in arriving at a suitable diagnosis. As for sugar, when I made my observation I knew absolutely nothing about the great hypoglycemia controversy—I knew nothing at all about blood sugar except that it had something to do with diabetes. It was only after noting that my seizures, blackouts, and episodes of dizziness and anxiety had abruptly become much worse during Christmas, and that the only thing really different about Christmas was that I was eating a far greater number of sugar-laden foods than usual, that I became curious enough about the possible effects of sugar to search for an informed book to see if sugar had ever been associated with troubles of the kind I was having. I discovered that it had, which led me to request the glucose tolerance test during which, as you know, all my worst symptoms were duplicated in the extreme. (See the following graph.)"

[*Note:* In interpreting blood glucose tests, physicians tend to set a "magic number," a sugar level above which you are normal, below which you are hypoglycemic. If you consider the graph which the professor is about to present in his letter (Figure 1), you will note his very severe symptoms at various stages of the test—though at no time were his sugar levels low enough to be called "hypoglyemic" by any of the "magic number" standards. Thus medical men miss an important point: a person with symptoms of low blood sugar is a person who can't stand small fluctuations in his blood sugar levels, although you and I may not be sensitive to them. The symptoms provoked by the test are meaningful; the numbers are not. Yet on the basis of such arbitrary "magic numbers," thousands of hypoglycemics—and I know whereof I write—have been told their tests were normal and their troubles "all in the mind." Which led, of course, to referral to psychiatrists for the couch, conversation, and calmative drugs. It has also led to dissatisfied psychiatrists, as well as patients, with the result that a number of these practitioners are now "orthomolecular"—using nutrition and nutrients to accomplish what they couldn't with tranquilizers, talk, antidepressants, and ECT (electroconvulsive or shock therapy).]

"Your second mistake," the professor continues, "especially in the light of the preceding, was in not questioning me about my dietary history. It would seem that some knowledge of a patient's food intake would be especially useful in diagnosing metabolic and endocrine abnormalities. *

"It was only after studying the literature on hypoglycemia that I realized that I had been exhibiting another classical symptom of hypoglycemia for many months, perhaps several years: a craving for sweets. I had developed a special affinity for chocolate, and was buying large economy boxes of Nestlé's Quik in order to save money on the two, three, and sometimes four large glasses of chocolate milk that seemed necessary before I could go to sleep at night. *

Urging more teaching of nutrition in medical schools, the professor offers to testify on the subject, and remarks: "In a medical problem involving food, it might well be that a more thorough knowledge of nutritional matters would provide a practical way around the miasma of confusion which presently characterizes endocrinological approaches to hypoglycemia and other nutrition-related disorders."

[*Note:* The professor's glucose tolerance test, Figure 1, was grossly misinterpreted at the ———— Hospital, a teaching institution associated with a major medical school. The test results were labeled "normal" although the patient was enduring a seizure, stuttering, and loss of color vision—all this a vivid example of the futility of diagnosing by the numbers alone. Ironically, in the year this test was given and misinterpreted at a famous hospital, the AMA announced that hypoglycemia is nonexistent, an imaginary disease.]

---

*The *Medical Tribune* of January 24, 1979, reports that six hospitals in ten do *not* routinely check the nutritional status of patients, and condemns the persistent administration of intravenous glucose. Can you imagine what happens to a hypoglycemic when he is pumped with sugar *intravenously*, as a substitute for food?

*A strong craving for chocolate, sugar, or any other food or beverage may indicate not only hypoglycemia but addictive allergy. It is analogous to the craving of the hard-drug addict who must obtain the next "fix" to stave off withdrawal symptoms.

The professor's letter to his doctor continues: "Your third and probably most serious mistake was in ignoring my violent reaction to the glucose, in insisting that my test was 'normal' in spite of the fact that I had a severe psychomotor seizure, probably at the onset of pancreatic activity, during which I shook convulsively, cried uncontrollably, could not hear or speak, and was finally rendered unconscious, after which I experienced episodes of stuttering and shaking at intervals of from five to ten minutes; then a period of extreme weakness and dizziness during which I could not walk to the water fountain without leaning against the wall.

"All of this happened within plain view of many technicians, lab workers, and receptionists, whom I requested that you speak with and whom you said you had. I myself reported the parts I could remember to you. I do not understand how you could regard my reaction to the test as 'normal,' or why when I was at last taken into the hospital on a stretcher a few weeks later one of your first actions was to place me on a 'normal' diet. The symptoms I manifested during this glucose tolerance test were the worst of those I had come to you complaining about; they were those of severe reactive hypoglycemia, and have been recognized as such since 1924 when Seale Harris first identified hyperinsulinism (overproduction of the hormone that recycles and 'burns' sugar) as a disease entity. One of the most comprehensive presentations of these symptoms remains the Seale Harris article. (See also two articles by Conn and Seltzer, and Hofeldt, Dippe, and Forsham.)

"The reason you interpreted the results of my test as 'normal' was, of course, that my blood glucose drop was above the 60 mg. point often used as a criterion for a diagnosis of possible hypoglycemia. But in the light of the widely varying interpretations which have been placed upon blood glucose values, it was definitely a mistake to trust these 'normal-range' figures in the face of the fact that my reactions to the sugar were anything but normal and all occurred within the spectrum of pancreatic activity and associated counterregulatory mechanisms."

The professor next discusses highly technical comments in various scientific papers dealing with the error in the "magic number" definition of low blood sugar. He concludes: "Fabrykant has concluded that reactive hypoglycemia results from an abnormal 'reaction threshold' to blood glucose variations rather than from low blood sugar itself, and he believes that the reproduction of the patient's symptoms while he is undergoing the glucose tolerance test is the single most reliable indicator of probable hypoglycemia.

"Your next mistake was in not hospitalizing me for observation immediately following my glucose tolerance test, not keeping me on a strict hypoglycemia diet with bed rest and a tranquilizer, and not providing me with sychiatric counseling by someone who knew what I had and the psychological disturbances that accompany it."

I omit several more highly technical paragraphs, in themselves a tribute to the determination of a medically untrained person to master a problem in medical nutrition, which he did. He then comments bitterly on hospital procedures and diet, none of them soothing for a hypoglycemic:

"Whether or not all this testing was necessary, it is clear that the absence of medication, the hurrying back and forth from X ray to brain scan to cardiology to EEG to inkblots, the incessant interviews, and the normal diet (coffee cake for breakfast, cobbler for lunch, ice cream for dinner) all aggravated my condition considerably. While the physical effects such as falling out of a wheelchair were bad enough, the most serious effects of all this were psychological. It is impossible to describe the feeling one has when he knows that he is physically ill, yet is being regarded as a lunatic by those entrusted with his care. And indeed I am sure that my morning seizures, the tears, the shaking, rolling back and forth, bawling out the nurses, staggering about the room, and saying incessantly that the room was moving in one direction while I was moving in another did appear rather strange. The mistake here, which I consider extremely serious, was that my illness was interpreted as psychosomatic rather than somatopsychic. I kept trying to tell you that I was *sick*, and that my pains and problems were extremely real, and you wrote off my sickness as 'subjective.' I suppose that I should be happy that my

37

eyes crossed so that you could at last have something to measure, although for me this was merely the last in a series of horrors, some of which were indescribable."

After some discussion of psychological testing which reveals that all hypoglycemics score abnormally high for hysteria and hypochondriasis (with an overemphasis on "meaningless" symptoms which, of course, may be quite meaningful for people with low blood sugar), the professor levels his next indictment:

"Your next mistake, a logical extension of your diagnosis of psychosomatic illness, was sending me to a psychiatrist without telling him anything at all about the nature of my illness, my symptoms, or my hospitalization. And the psychiatrist obviously felt no need to know about any of these things either, since he made no attempt to find out about them. On my first visit, he simply escorted me into his office and sat down, saying nothing but, 'What are your thoughts?' Sizing up his method as totally nondirective, I obliged by talking for two months about anything psychological I could think of, dragging out whatever skeletons I could remember from the closets of my childhood and adolescence. All these had seen the light of day many times before, and none was especially painful to look at again. I was presuming, of course, that the psychiatrist was measuring what I was saying against the kind of illness I presumed he knew I had, and I was frankly infuriated when I discovered, almost by accident, that he knew nothing about why I had come to him. This entire episode constituted an enormous waste of time, money, and effort and contributed nothing but increased stress and fatigue to the process of my recovery. Ironically, the only clearly 'neurotic' tendency he as able, apparently, to discern was—surprise—a congenital inability to place implicit trust in authority figures. Now, I wonder what kinds of experiences over the past few years could possibly have confirmed in me the opinion that authority figures could not always be trusted?"

The educator closes with several requests and two demands, aware that some of them will seem outrageous: "1. I would like a complete review of my case by all of those who participated in it. I would like the facts presented as they are . . . and the diagnosis changed from 'psychosomatic illness' to 'severe reactive hypoglycemia with cerebral complications' or something to that effect."

[*Note:* To this day—these lines are written in February 1979—some hospitals are known to refuse to admit patients with a diagnosis of functional or reactive hypoglycemia, and Blue Cross has been (successfully) sued because it refused to pay bills for treatment of the disorder. Who admits or pays for treatment of patients with an imaginary disease?]

"2. I would like the fruits of this review presented in a Grand Rounds session. . . . Those bewildered residents, interns, nurses, and aides who saw me performing my stunts every day need to know exactly what it was they were witnessing.

"3. I demand that you carefully *watch* patients undergoing the glucose tolerance test for the classical symptoms of reactive hypoglycemia, and that you hospitalize immediately those whose reactions are severe and give them appropriate treatment, all of this completely without regard for the particular points within the spectrum of pancreatic activity at which these symptoms appear." [In other words, drop the "magic number" philosophy.]

"4. I demand that you review the medical records of every patient you and the other clinic doctors have consigned to the psychiatric ward of ———— and ———— hospitals, screening for possible hypoglycemics. I demand that those who manifest hypoglycemic symptoms be given a glucose tolerance test, and that those who show a drop from fasting level exceeding 20 mg. percent or whose symptoms are markedly aggravated by the glucose be placed immediately on the hypoglycemia diet. Hypoglycemia can drive one crazy, and judging from your handling of my case, I think there is a good possibility that you have missed quite a few of us."

[*Note:* A friend of mine, an Ohio psychiatrist, long ago demonstrated that patients in any psychiatric practice may include many hypoglycemics whose physical disease has not been recognized although it has aggravated—if not initiated—their troubles. When he called back patients he had previously discharged who had been treated for "purely psychiatric" disorders, he found

60 percent of them to be hypoglycemics, which meant they had troubles which weren't helped for want of competent diagnosis and treatment.]

The professor asked his physician to write a letter to me, since it was my book which led his patient to correct diagnosis and treatment of his low blood sugar. He asked the doctor to detail the case from his own perspective so that this history, as I have presented it to you, might be "as informed and balanced as possible." The doctor agreed to do so, but I never heard from him.

The professor's last statement is remarkable for two reasons: (1) it contains the equally impassioned outcry of a physician, Dr. Stephen Gyland, who himself was a hypoglycemic and endured the gratuitous tortures against which the educator is protesting. Ironically, this account was published in the *Journal of the American Medical Association (JAMA)*, the publication of the medical establishment which had warned physicians that competent doctors don't treat hypoglycemia, the "nondisease." Quoting Dr. Gyland, the professor concludes:

" 'If all physicians would read the work of Dr. Seale Harris . . . thousands of persons would not have to go through what I did. During three years of severe illness I was examined by fourteen specialists and three nationally known clinics before a diagnosis [of hypoglycemia] was made by means of a six-hour glucose tolerance test, previous diagnoses having been brain tumor, diabetes, and cerebral arteriosclerosis. . . . Regardless of the outcome of the glucose tolerance test, hypoglycemic symptoms call for a trial of the diet anyway, and if hypoglycemia is the problem, improvement with the proper diet should be spectacular in one or two weeks.' " To which the educator tersely adds: "It was."

I was aware of Dr. Gyland's fiery indictment of the medical blindness to hypoglycemia long before the professor encountered it. The Gyland story even has a sardonic twist: after the physician had recovered, thanks to the Seale Harris diet, he specialized in hypoglycemia, treating more than 1,100 patients, all hypoglycemics, all previously victims of faulty diagnoses. Dr. Gyland then wrote a fascinating paper on his 1,100 rescuees—and couldn't persuade any U.S. medical journal to publish it. So it was that, searching for the Gyland paper in vain, I finally obtained a copy through his family—published in Brazil, in Portuguese.

If you think my friend the professor managed to develop uniquely bizarre symptoms deriving from his low blood sugar, it will be very instructive to study the list of symptoms Gyland recorded in his 1,100 sufferers. Figure 2 shows what percentage of the patients complained of each particular symptom.

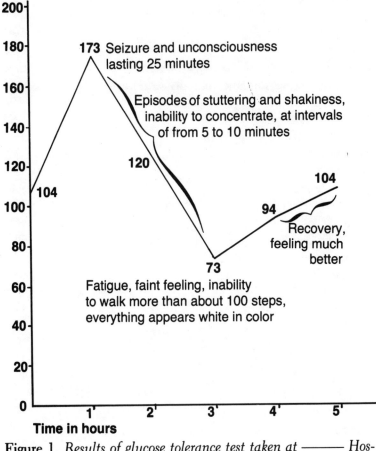

Figure 1. *Results of glucose tolerance test taken at* ——— *Hospital, January 1974. Results interpreted as "normal."*

Figure 2. *Symptoms complained of by patients of Dr. Stephen Gyland, with percentages of patients complaining of each.*

Nervousness	94%
Irritability	89%
Exhaustion	87%
Faintness, dizziness, tremor, cold sweats, weak spells	86%
Depression	77%
Vertigo, dizziness	73%
Drowsiness	72%
Headaches	71%
Digestive disturbances	69%
Forgetfulness	67%
Constant worrying, unprovoked anxieties	62%
Insomnia (awakening and inability to return to sleep)	62%
Internal trembling	57%
Mental confusion	57%
Palpitation of heart, rapid pulse	54%
Muscle pains	53%
Numbness	51%
Indecisiveness	50%
Unsocial, asocial, antisocial behavior	47%
Crying spells	46%
Lack of sex drive (females)	44%
Allergies	43%
Incoordination	43%
Leg cramps	43%
Lack of concentration	42%
Blurred vision	40%
Twitching and jerking of muscles	40%
Itching and crawling sensations on skin	39%
Gasping for breath	37%
Smothering spells	34%
Staggering	34%
Sighing and yawning	30%
Impotence (males)	29%
Night terrors, nightmares	27%

Unconsciousness	27%
Rheumatoid arthritis	24%
Phobias, fears	23%
Neurodermatitis	21%
Suicidal intent	20%
Nervous breakdown	17%
Convulsions	2%

The patients also commented on changes in personality in the form of unaccustomed lapses in moral conduct, carelessness in dress, and tendencies to drug and alcohol addiction.

Look back over that list of symptoms. How could these patients have convinced any physician that they weren't neurotics?

A large percentage of them *had* been told that their symptoms were expressions of neurotic conflicts. Here are some of the mistaken diagnoses they received before Dr. Gyland subjected them to the simple but time-consuming sugar-tolerance test:

Mental Retardation

Neurosis

"Slightly nervous"

Chronic urticaria (hives)

Neurodermatitis (itching, rash, from "nervous" causes)

Menière's syndrome (loss of hearing, dizziness associated with it, and noises in the ears)

Cerebral arteriosclerosis

Cephalalgia, hemicrania (pain in the head, or in half the head)

Psychoneuroticism

Chronic bronchial asthma

Rheumatoid arthritis

Parkinson's syndrome (senile palsy)

Paroxysmal tachycardia (rapid beating of the heart)

"Imaginary sickness"

Menopause

Alcoholism

Diabetes

Hyperinsulinism (the correct diagnosis—but treated with candy bars!)

43

Notes from the Nutritionist's Diary

In 1924 Dr. Seale Harris published the paper first recognizing low blood sugar. It appeared in *JAMA*. Since medical indifference to—or denial of the existence of—hypoglycemia persists to this day, one might wonder if there is anything intrinsic to medical thinking that automatically makes new ideas suspect, even when they're fifty years old. Apparently there is, and it creates a cultural lag which is the despair of the young physician and a totally frustrating experience for those patients who seek alternative and more effective tests and treatments. But cultural lag isn't a phenomenon of the medical mind alone. Recently, on the *60-Minutes* CBS TV program, we watched a child visibly suffering from the symptoms of withdrawal from sugar. That was preceded by a eulogy of sugared foods by a Harvard nutritionist (whose department is heavily subsidized by manufacturers of such nonfoods) and followed by a bland statement from an officer of a giant manufacturer of sweetened cereals who had seen the child's suffering but insisted that, nonetheless, sugar and sugared cereals are an unmitigated boon to the young.

Since I published *Low Blood Sugar and You* there have been developments which negate some of the frustration I felt—and you must have felt—in reading the letters in this chapter. Many of the younger physicians are fully aware of hypoglycemia, do test for it, do successfully treat it, and thereby invite the censure of the medical establishment. A spate of books on low blood sugar has descended on the public. Some of them are useful, and some record the authors' personal theories which collide with hard-won clinical fact. A typical claim has it that high-protein diets for hypoglycemia are "old-fashioned." I have no time for debate, but will point out that the letters you have just read all came from people whose problems with hypoglycemia were solved by the "old-fashioned" high-protein diet, and those communications are but a sampling of tens of thousands I've received. Maybe they had old-fashioned hypoglycemia? I don't know, but I do know that generalizations in nutrition are untrustworthy. Many patients thrive on high-protein, high-fat, low-carbohydrate diets; some need other types. Jack Spratt does exist, and our biochemical differences are greater than our similarities.

Postdating my hypoglycemia book by some ten years, this chapter gives me a chance to reemphasize some of the important points about low blood sugar, a few of them only recently come by:

1. We really should not perform glucose tolerance tests. They can be misleading. For example, there is a small amount of corn protein in glucose, and an adverse reaction blamed on the sugar might instead result from allergy to corn. The test is a highly artificial construct anyway: a large dose of sugar on an empty stomach, with or without adverse reactions, doesn't tell us much about the patient's tolerance for other foods. And other foods may play hob with blood glucose stability too. In fact, allergy to a food can raise the blood sugar in diabetes, lower it in hypoglycemics, or cause all the symptoms of low blood sugar with no change in blood glucose levels. A sensible alternative to the glucose tolerance test is to check your blood sugar before and after your usual breakfast in midmorning, before and after lunch, and in midafternoon. Now we are studying you, not in the sterile atmosphere of a laboratory after a synthetic "meal" of processed glucose, but as you normally (or abnormally) live and as you normally (abnormally) eat.

2. Keep a double diary: everything you eat or drink and the times when, plus a list of every symptom, major or minor. The doctor who understands hypoglycemia will not consider you a hypochondriac for this. He will find it invaluable in tracing what in your diet is disturbing the wisdom of the body.

3. If you're on the hypoglycemia diet and still have difficulty in starting your day, try rising earlier, having an earlier breakfast, and going back to bed for an hour. This sometimes helps to recharge the batteries.

4. Remember that frequent small meals help to stabilize blood sugar, cholesterol, and weight. Larger meals, even though the day's food total is the same, do the opposite.

5. The supplements your doctor prescribes are not optional. As I've noted, the liver is important in regulation of sugar metabolism, and supplements in hypoglycemia are aimed in part at helping liver function and at oxidation (burning) of sugar and

starches. This is particularly pertinent to the Vitamin B Complex and desiccated liver supplements.

6. In some hypoglycemics, probably the majority, the adrenal glands are in trouble because they are faced with the task of raising the blood sugar when the overactive pancreas is busy trying excessively to lower it. When the sugar-free diet quiets down the pancreas, the adrenal glands can then function normally and need no further help. But in some patients the adrenals are in direct failure and remain so even when the pancreas is no longer overactive. This explains your physician's use of adrenal cortex injections. He is trying to give your adrenal glands a little rest by supplying the hormones from an external source. As part of the battle to have hypoglycemics competently diagnosed and treated, there is an effort on the part of the Food and Drug Administration, acting on AMA philosophy, to ban the use of adrenal cortex injections in the treatment of hypoglycemia. We anticipate that with the help of congressmen and senators, already offered, we may be able to persuade the FDA that there is no room for a government agency in the practice of medicine or, more particularly, in the intimate relationship between the competent medical nutritionist and his informed patient.

7. Your doctor may give you a supplement of glycerin. This is used because it is converted into glycogen (*stored* sugar) which, not directly entering the blood, builds your reserves so that you can draw upon them when in need.

8. Avocado contains an odd type of sugar which not only doesn't stimulate the production of insulin by the pancreas but depresses it. Fine for hypoglycemics, but not for diabetics.

9. Clues to the start of hypoglycemia may be found in a family history of diabetes or allergy or both. Environmental causes include the psychic (largely in a feeling of lack of accomplishment and recognition) and the dietetic (poor nutrition, particularly when aggravated by excessive use of sugar, coffee, tea, chocolate, and cola beverages). Stress, as you have learned, often lights the fuse.

Mentioning glycerin reminds me of another story. This time the protagonists were a medical man and his nutritionist patient (myself). I had stopped in for a genitourinary checkup, on the same trip to California where I met the recovered alcoholic whose letter you read earlier in this chapter. When the GU specialist discovered my professsion, he announced that he suffered from reactive hypoglycemia. If he ate breakfast, he told me, his blood sugar dropped so low that he couldn't see clearly and was likely to walk into a wall when seeking a doorway. For that reason, he added, he no longer ate breakfast. I suggested that surrendering to the metabolic storm wasn't particularly good medicine or, for that matter, good nutrition, and gave him notes about the Vitamin B Complex, the low-sugar, high-protein diet, the frequent small meals, and the use of a supplement of glycerin.

When I returned early one morning for the results of my tests, he was reading a medical journal. The blurring and the incoordination were gone, he said, and thanked me. When I asked for my bill, he smiled and said it was a Mexican standoff. "Who consulted with whom?" he asked, and refused to allow me to pay. When I got home I sent him my text on low blood sugar, suitably autographed, I thought, since he was a kidney-bladder expert: "From an expert in input to an expert in output."

3
Nutrition and Disorders "of the Mind"

My Pixie Wife, Betty, and I were visiting the rug department of a neighborhood department store where, happily, the saleswoman didn't recognize me. (Many listeners and readers in our home area do, and it always means a barrage of questions about nutrition. In fact, I once remarked that the only time I was ever late for a broadcast was when I met a neighbor and asked her how she was—and she told me.)

The saleswoman asked my Pixie Wife for our address, not our name: she was merely arranging to have the rug area in our home measured. She stared at the address and remarked, "You must live near Carlton Fredericks." My P.W., with a straight face, replied, "He's practically on top of me." That, of course, was lost on the saleswoman, who continued: "I saw him on the Merv Griffin show on TV, and I fell in love with him. But he did seem a little arrogant." "He's the worst," said my P.W. with a straight face. "I slept with him the other night, and he didn't even say thank you!" "It shows you," said the woman with conviction, "that you can judge a person by watching him on television." Then she asked for the name, and my P.W. said, "Betty Fredericks." It still didn't register. Not until we were walking away did we hear a long scream followed by, "I feel so *stupid!*"

Hindsight is 20–20, but it sometimes makes me feel myopic. I'm thinking of research a physician and I conducted with a group of "delinquent" children, in which we showed there was much more and severer allergy in these children than one would find in the normal child population. We were led to ponder the tendency of delinquent children to develop allergies, but we never thought of the possibility that allergy made them delinquent. Allergists then didn't recognize, and I certainly didn't, that the brain isn't immune to allergic reactions which can alter behavior, with results which may be socially unacceptable or medically pathological. And allergy is only one small aspect of the relationships among foods, neurosis, psychosis, autism, hyperactivity, and asocial behavior. Some of the case histories in my diary perfectly illustrate that interplay.

A Canadian correspondent, who wrote that his radio blurred and he couldn't catch my name, addressed a letter to me as "The Hypoglycemia Specialist," New York City, and it reached me at New York's station WOR on which I've broadcast for some fifteen years. (Explanation: I have a number of listeners and readers in the main New York post office. They tune in while eating hero sandwiches, washed down with Cokes.)

The Canadian listener's letter is an eloquent description of cerebral allergy, unrecognized for years. He wrote: "One sleepless night, I tuned in to WOR and heard you say that hypoglycemia could be caused by a food allergy. For years, I had suffered from constant fatigue, chronic headaches, sleeplessness, and was never free from aches and pains. I was so weary and unable to cope that I no longer cared if I lived or died. The next morning, I went off all wheat products. All my symptoms disappeared, and I'm like a new person, thanks to you—you saved my life!"

The letter arrived a week before *The New York Times* science reporter announced that hypoglycemia is an imaginary disease. Next, probably, they'll get around to a similar classification for cerebral allergy.

Other pages in my diary are devoted to Elise, a paranoid schizophrenic who heard voices which twice forced her to set fire to her parents' home. The barrage of drugs her psychiatrist pre-

49

scribed softened but didn't completely still what she called "the anvil chorus" in her head. Her besetting nutritional sin was chocolate, for which she had a compulsion reminiscent of the inexorable craving of the heroin addict. So pronounced an addiction is a red flag to the nutritionist who is aware that we are often addicted to the very foods to which we are most allergic. The process is strikingly like that in those who are hooked on hard drugs. Their craving is not only for the "high" but also for protection from the withdrawal symptoms, and both the stimulation and the withdrawal symptoms can be reactions to consuming—or deserting—a food to which we are allergic.

We were able to demonstrate that avoiding chocolate was an important key to sanity for Elise. Whenever she complained again of the subjective voices, she would ultimately confess that she had weakened and eaten a "little chocolate," which could have been anything from a single cookie to a full pound of candy. In Elise's case, we were able to find a "neutralizing dose," a minute and precise amount of chocolate, dissolved in a full glass of water, which significantly eased both the craving and the withdrawal symptoms. We believe it fools the brain into the belief that the craving has been satisfied—a poor and unscientific explanation, but Elise and her parents (who can now all sleep peacefully) don't care.

There is no way, unless you've seen the effects, for an average person to imagine the impact of the "wrong molecules" on the brain. My diary carries a memo on "caffeine madness." It is the history of a schizophrenic young man whose mother rewarded him for good behavior by giving him cola drinks. She couldn't be persuaded that for him caffeine and sugar were molecules of madness. His psychiatrist had deserted couch and tranquilizer "treatment" in favor of the biochemical, which proved the patient's salvation. The physician taped an interview with the patient, who was accompanied, on the practitioner's insistence, by his mother. During what to that point had been a coherent conversation, the physician gave the patient a full glass of Coca-Cola. Over a period of about twenty minutes the patient's remarks slowly became an inaudible murmur. He slipped from the chair, lay on the floor in the fetal position with his thumb in his mouth, and screamed for his mother—who was kneeling beside him. As you listen to the tape, you hear her plead with him, and then there is an agonized cry: "Oh, God! I didn't realize what I was doing to my boy." That was followed by the patient's slow return to sanity, following a neutralizing dose of cola accompanied by a massive injection of Vitamin C and Vitamin B_6.

It should be noted that the American Psychiatric Association pronounces this kind of treatment valueless in schizophrenia. They base their authoritative statement on an experiment in which they tested the wrong vitamin in the wrong dose on the wrong type of patient, under the direction of a psychiatric committee which included one practitioner who was on the payroll of a tranquilizer company and another who admitted he was entering the project with the conviction that the treatment would be proved to be quackery. The report, nonetheless, is cited by practitioners who deny the validity of a biochemical approach to mental disease. But what is it they are doing when they prescribe tranquilizers and antidepressants?

Although paranoid behavior is considered by cynics to be normal in married men, it is a frequent aspect of schizophrenia. My diary records the story of a schizophrenic mother with elaborate delusions of persecution, both of whose children showed ominous symptoms of the disorder. The smaller boy heard voices addressing him from the clouds, and his older brother talked each night with his grandfather, long deceased, who appeared in his bedroom as a "purple cloud." A geneticist would have had a field day with a family that so beautifully illustrated the power of a few aberrant chromosomes. A behavioral psychiatrist would have made it a strong case for environmental influences in this common mental disorder. A bioecological allergist came up with the real answer when he insisted that wheat be withdrawn from the family diet; it was, and the symptoms swiftly disappeared. You might logically wonder what made the allergist suspicious of an impact of wheat allergy on the brain, but it was no wild stab. During World War II, shortage of shipping created a shortage of wheat in blockaded countries ordinarily consuming large amounts of bread. During that period, admissions of schizo-phrenics to hospitals fell off sharply. Following that clue, an American psychiatrist withdrew wheat from the diets of institu-tionalized schizophrenics and observed substantial improvement. The corollary also proved true: restoring wheat to the diet, in capsule form so that the patients were not aware of its reintro-duction, aggravated the schizophrenic symptoms and negated much of the small benefits the patients had received from med-ication. In my diary, I appended a note of frustration: to this day, more than thirty years after the war, bread and wheat products are the "staff of psychosis" in the kitchens of practically all es-tablishment mental institutions.

In the 1960s, I was approached in Miami Beach by a woman who obviously expected me to recognize her. When I pleaded that I couldn't possibly remember the tens of thousands of people I've met in a long career in public life, she said: "But you pho-tographed me in the nude!" I gave the only possible response: "Take your clothes off!" Before you conclude that I was an early arrival on the pornographic scene, let me explain that Dr. Harry Swartz and I were conducting an experiment in which we used vitamin and other supplements to redistribute body fat toward the normal. We were particularly interested in the problem areas—those which tenaciously retain fat deposits despite weight loss—and we had some success. One elderly women who had volunteered for the research wasn't successful in changing her figure, but did send me a note which emphasizes the dividends that accrue from a favorable change in the biochemistry of the brain: "I don't know what you gave us," she confessed, "but there must have been something which, with all the supplements I've used, I never took before. It fell upon me as a blanket of peace." The date was 1962. The agent of peacefulness was lecithin. In 1978, an M.I.T. research team announced a great stride in nu-tritional modification of neurotransmitters in the brain achieved with—what else?—lecithin. They found it helped both the senile and the normal particularly with reference to memory.

Over the years I fought an unremitting battle with the food establishment and its captive professors at the universities heavily subsidized by its grants. So it is that my diary tells the story of a crying schoolteacher—surely a subject which doesn't seem capable of igniting a battle between Harvard University and one small nutritionist, but it did. The teacher was in her sixties and nearing retirement. She feared she would be retired prematurely and would lose some of her pension because of her unprovoked weeping, which frequently occurred in the classroom. She was herself oblivious to these attacks, which startled the children into nervous laughter, until a complaint came from the mother of one of her pupils. She then wrote to me, pleading for reference to a psychiatrist, but I detoured her to a medical nutritionist. I wasn't being arbitrary: every competent worker in my field is (or should be) aware that niacinamide deficiency will cause not only "swimmy-headedness" but loss of a sense of humor and "weepiness." A few injections of the vitamin were accompanied by oral doses of the entire Vitamin B Complex, since deficiency in just one of these vitamins, which appear in foods together, is unlikely. She made it a point at one of my university seminars to identify herself as the "formerly crying schoolteacher." A Harvard professor used valuable space in his syndicated nutrition feature to denounce the story as "nonsense." I didn't bother to supply him with the scientific references which document inexplicable crying as a possible early symptom of deficiency in niacinamide, feeling that only a sizable grant to his department would be effective in correcting his thinking.

At the time this minor battle was being fought, I was under attack by the FDA as a "food faddist," defined as anyone who is un-American enough to criticize white bread, sugar, and cornflakes. One of my public relations people bearded the FDA lion by lunching with the then commissioner of that agency and suggesting that he have a chat with me. The commissioner reeled under the impact of the proposal. "I will *not!*" he blurted. My PR man wanted to know why the suggestion was so outrageous. "The son of a bitch," was the candid reply, "might convince me that we're wrong." I gave a page in the diary to that admission.

Sometimes the physical universe can suddenly become unstable and realities can change unpredictably. If you're aware of it and can do nothing about it, you're likely to grope for the couch of the nearest psychiatrist. One student who had these frightening encounters with a world gone beserk didn't—he was too terrified. Instead, he locked himself in his bedroom and refused to leave it, offering no explanation to his wife. She never explained what intuition made her take him to an orthomolecular psychiatrist, but she did, and he found himself in a laboratory undergoing a number of blood tests. Only one of the vitamin levels was low, and that was in the normal range. But the physician knew, as all health professionals must learn, that "low normal" for *you* may not be adequate, and on that slender premise he gave the student a series of Vitamin B_{12} injections. The vitamin, ordinarily used for the prevention and treatment of pernicious anemia, had no apparent effect until the third week of treatment, and then the symptoms gradually faded. They had included apparent lengthening and shortening of streets, buildings growing taller and shorter, peoples' faces ballooning and shrinking, and the patient's own hands appearing to change in size. To keep reality at bedrock stability, he must have the injections every third day, which is interesting because an injection of the vitamin "wears off" at about that interval.

The student's history is reminiscent of another, that of an elderly woman patient who had been brought to a sanitarium for shock therapy for "senile paranoid dementia," or second childhood with delusions of persecution. Something made the psychiatrist feel that her illness had nothing to do with the aging process, and his tests confirmed that her nervous system was physically deteriorating because of a deficiency in Vitamin B_{12}, although she didn't show the anemia typical of that disease. Prior to treatment her paranoid delusion was severe (she accused her husband of trying to irradiate her when he moved the television set nearer her bed), but she left the institution a normal human being.

Long before my friend, that towering genius Linus Pauling, had coined the term "orthomolecular," I had—and missed—the opportunity to initiate the concept. My diary relates the story of a woman who was being treated for functional gallbladder syndrome—meaning that there were as yet no gallstones to force surgery. She had other troubles of which I wasn't aware until, while discussing her new diet and supplements with her, I was suddenly confronted with a full-fledged delusion of persecution. She said she would have trouble following the new diet because "there are men following me, trying to poison me, so I have to buy all my foods in sealed packages." I quieted her by reminding her that she was in the hands of caring professionals, and proceeded to set up the program of controlled diet and supplements, aimed primarily at liver function, which is more involved in gallbladder syndrome than is recognized even to this day. After a few months of augmented intake of the B vitamins plus desiccated liver, and with improvement in her tolerance for fats and fiber, she spontanously remarked: "I don't see those men anymore. They must be hiding." Two months after that, I asked her about the men who were trying to poison her. "What men?" she asked, genuinely convinced that I had lost my mind. The diary entry came back to my memory in full detail when I heard some orthomolecular psychiatrists reporting on the improvement in paranoid schizophrenics given the benefit of massive doses of the B vitamins, but that was twenty years later.

It was only a few years after his colleagues contemptuously rejected Smith Ely Jellife's concept of the psychosomatic that it became difficult to persuade physicians that your illness was not "all in your mind." The pendulum swung so far that, as Emmanuel Cheraskin has remarked, it became possible to be "treated" with conversation and calmative drugs while suffering from an unrecognized brain tumor, which is to say that the overemphasis on the psychosomatic has led to neglect of the somatopsychic—the influence of body on mind. This is painfully apparent when one visits the institutions for the senile aged. There the emphasis is on the purely custodial, and *rehabilitation* is an empty word. How do you rehabilitate a mind impaired by hardening of the arteries? Answer: sometimes you can, if you practice holistic psychiatry, medicine, or nutrition. In my diary, I am reminded of a nursing home where I encountered a ninety-four-year-old lawyer. He was neatly dressed but silent, obviously listening to the beat of a distant drum. As I came into the sanitarium he was seated in a chair facing the doorway, his eyes unfocused, oblivious to his surroundings. As the medical man who owned the institution had requested, I revised the diets of his patients and installed a large bottle of Vitamin B Complex syrup in the pharmacy, which eliminated the morning lineup for laxatives. To selected patients, among them the aged lawyer, we gave supplements of glutamine, Vitamin E, and Vitamin B Complex by injection. When I returned to the home about six months later, the ninety-four-year-old was seated in the same chair, facing the door. He was reading *The New York Times.* This could be interpreted as a relapse, of course, but I harbor no animosity against a faithful voice of establishment medicine.

Many of the older people who are relegated to the scrap heap of senility display symptoms, readily apparent to the trained eye, of nutritional deficiencies. Correcting them doesn't always restore the aged to social and vocational usefulness, but sometimes it does, and in any case the patients at least feel and function a little better. This improvement is not always appreciated by the family, for I have a diary note on a totally unexpected response from the wife of an old man who had been brought back to reality by nutritional therapies. She confronted me at the sanitarium with: "He asked me about the business, and the bank balances, and he wants to see the checkbooks. I don't know what you're doing to him—but stop it!"

There is a "Social Security" level of nutritional deficiency which, like the income from the government, doesn't license death and doesn't permit living. A victim of this was Millie, who was thirty-one years old and had been sick for thirty-one years. She was a patient at the Shaler Lawton Foundation, where I supervised the nutrition department. Her internist asked that her diet be altered to minimize, if possible, the constant gastric pain she patiently endured. Indeed, her diet history was a tribute to the ability of the body to accommodate to long-term borderline deficiencies. That was what made me react sharply when she told me that she always felt "swimmy-headed." (I mentioned this symptom earlier as a frequent byproduct of a diet low in niacinamide.) Originally, the condition was mentioned in a lecture by Dr. Tom Spies, a medical nutritionist famous for his research in the early or so-called "preclinical" symptoms of the penalties for a diet neither good enough to support health nor bad enough to precipitate outright, "classical" deficiency symptoms. All this means that Millie's "swimmy-headedness" could have been a prelude to the delirium which pellagra can cause. (Its other symptoms are diarrhea and dermatitis—hence it's the disease of the "three *d's*.")

I advised the physician that I was placing her on high-protein foods supplemented with a Vitamin B Complex concentrate, brewer's yeast, and extra niacinamide. She came to see me a few weeks later with a report which managed to leave me both happy and depressed. "I'm thinking normally," she said, "maybe for the first time in my life. I told that to Doctor ———, and he said that was fine—and I should stop taking the vitamins." To the internist, in protest, I quoted Dr. Spies, who said that nutritional therapy must be consistent, comprehensive, concentrated, and continuous. So was the internist's rejection of the whole idea.

Actually, I wasn't struggling with him as a person but with the time-dishonored resistance of medicine to new ideas. After all, Spies' observations were only twenty years old at the time. And if my patience impresses you, don't let it. I still writhe when I remember that in the 1940s a large cancer society cancelled a citation intended for the emphasis I gave in my broadcasts on the value of frequent physical examinations for early detection of cancer. Their reason: I was giving the public "false hope" by linking nutrition with cancer. That was fascinating for two reasons. First, the information I gave in the context of nutrition versus cancer, came from a monograph published by the New York Academy of Sciences. And now, more than thirty years later, that same cancer society is emphasizing good nutrition as a means of reducing the incidence of the disease.

One may hope that the resistance of pediatricians to the nutritional treatment of hyperactive children will follow the same pattern, maybe a little more expeditiously. It isn't comforting that

57

the Academy of Pediatrics recently announced that diets free of additives might inflict who knows what consequences on the children. It is a little difficult to anticipate what harm might come to children deprived of Cokes, candy, sugar, coal-tar dyes, and Twinkies. But it is easy, if one is objective, to learn what benefit accrues to some children who are not permitted to consume these triumphs of modern food technology. The letter which follows is one of hundreds I've received which found its way to my diary, not only because it emphasizes the importance of controlled nutrition for some children who are hyperactive or who have learning problems, but because it is so heartwarming:

Writing from a small town in Canada, a mother pleaded for help. "We heard one of your broadcasts, and wished to write to you immediately, but didn't know your full name until having heard you again. Your first program that we heard dealt with orthomolecular psychiatry and Vitamin B_3 deficiency. You described symptoms a child may display in schoolwork. You were describing our daughter—i.e., poor attention span, apparent laziness, breaks in her memory pattern, hyperactivity, muscular coordination problems. After hearing the program and the indictment of food additives for their effect on some of these children, we put her on natural foods as much as possible. There was an immediate improvement in her schoolwork and she finished her school year successfully, whereas in February, she had sat the entire month accomplishing nothing.

"We took her to a mental health clinic for testing in May and June. She was revealed to be, I quote: 'A child of superior intelligence, but with a pronounced visual handicap and a muscular coordination difficulty.'

"Visual testing," the mother continued, "revealed that patterns normally seen on a horizontal plane appeared perpendicular to that line when viewed by our child. The clinic suggested additional work to be done in the school by the specialist there, perhaps an hour daily, and every effort was made by her classroom teacher to present an uncluttered visual field. I have worked at home with our daughter from Primary to Grade Eleven, both winter and summer, to help her keep up with her class.

"She tested extremely high in reading, and was above her grade level in most of her schoolwork but average in math. The greatest difficulty lies in math in shapes and patterns, and in reader workbook in arranging in alphabetical sequence as well as sentences in proper sequence.

"Since listening to the broadcasts in March and July, I feel our daughter could be helped by a correct diet. She appears to have suffered brain damage or has inherited a genetic disorder, causing her to be labeled as having a learning disability. . . . Her memory break seems to be greatly improved since removal of food additives in March.

"We would appreciate any information you could give us to help our daughter. E. and N. K."

This letter, with its information concerning food additives, was received about a year ago. During the period covered in the letter, the Journal of the American Medical Association announced that food additives have no deleterious effect on children. A year later, however, a paper reported in the same journal that erythrosin B, which is Red #3, used in candy, puddings, frosting, and cookies, becomes toxic when those who consume it are exposed to light. Sunbathers were given as an example. In that year, I received a paper from Dr. Stephen Kon, of the chemistry staff of New York's Mount Sinai Hospital, urging the use of this "FDA certified" food coloring as an insecticide to kill flies breeding in manure piles.

Meanwhile, Food and Drug Administration calculations indicate that a twelve-year-old child may already have eaten as much as three pounds of these dyes derived from coal tar. There are six of them, including Red #3, which have been "permanently" approved by FDA as safe. They include Citrus Red 2, which the World Health Organization labeled as cancer-producing in 1969. Blue #1, used in beverages, candy, and baked goods, is banned in Great Britain as a cancer producer. Orange B, used in hot dogs and sausage skins, is suspected of causing cancer, as is Red #3. Yellow #5, of which the public swallows thousands of pounds, creates serious allergic reactions in the sensitive, and has been indicted by Dr. Ben F. Feingold as an offender for hyperactive children. I find it less than comforting to know that the FDA joins the AMA in protecting us from the "food faddists" who criticize additives.

The letter from the Canadian mother is one of tens of thousands which cascade on my hapless if nutritious head. What can one do for her? Most correspondents in the United States have access to qualified bioecological allergists, even if not in their home areas, and to orthomolecular psychiatrists and internists. But in a small Canadian town, what chance will she have of locating a practitioner abreast of this avant-garde science? You may ask why I could not send her explicit guidance, to which there is an explicit answer: instruction in nutrition for a physical or mental problem is counted as the practice of medicine, and I am a Ph.D., not permitted so to prescribe. I should know: this ploy was used by the medical establishment in an effort to silence my broadcasts; they labeled my recommendation of a multiple-vitamin–mineral supplement, available at supermarkets, as the practice of medicine.

Instead, I sent the Canadian mother a copy of one of my books devoted to nutrition and the mind. In it there is a chapter which discusses control of the diet for the hyperactive, autistic, schizophrenic, "brain-damaged" children and for those with learning problems. I then referred her to a qualified practitioner in a larger Canadian city, which meant a long but, I was sure, worthwhile journey for the family. Having done what I could, I entered these notes in my diary, and went on to the next letter, and the next, and the next. They come in at the rate of nearly a thousand a day, half of them complaining, "I wrote to you the day before yesterday, and I haven't heard yet."

Months later, a note arrived from Canada, bubbling with the family's happiness. One paragraph gives the story's happy ending:

"Our daughter never felt confident enough to join in after-school play and social activities with her peers. Last night she stopped at the door, en route to a scout meeting at our church, her eyes dancing, to tell us again how much better she feels. God bless you and all those who carry on your work."

I put that in my diary, too. It's followed by this note: "The pediatric academy has come out in favor of breastfeeding. Now about those yellow cupcakes and Cokes. . . ."

Several of my notes deal with influences on the mind which are so subtle that they are never suspected, and frequently the end of the story is years of psychoanalysis or psychotherapy or an endless tide of tranquilizer and antidepressant prescriptions. There is the story of a woman who was depressed from the day she moved into a house she had inherited from her mother. What fodder for an analyst—the house was obviously a focal point for "unresolved conflicts" in her relationship with her deceased parent, with guilt underlying the depression. So were the fumes from the gasoline evaporating from the carburetor of her car, kept in a garage directly under her bedroom. When, at the urging of a bioecological allergist, she parked her car in the street, the depression largely lifted. It disappeared completely when she reluctantly yielded to the allergist's advice and had her new plastic tiling removed from the kitchen. Like gasoline, it is ultimately of petroleum origin and had touched off her sensitivity to these hydrocarbons.

Solanine is a poison found in potatoes, particularly in those exposed to light, which is certainly true both of those on sale in your supermarkets and of those in the bins of the potato chip factories. Average yearly consumption of solanine from potatoes aggregates about 9.7 grams, a dose which taken all at once would kill a horse. We escape fatal poisoning because we ingest it very gradually, but the advocates of free use of food additives cite solanine as an example of the "natural poisons" in food which don't bother us, thereby justifying the addition of synthetic chemicals—preservatives, stabilizers, and colors—to our diets. The argument rests on several fallacies, an obvious one being the belief that the body will cope with new and unaccustomed poisons as efficiently as it handles those with which it has had millennia of experience. Second, many of the natural poisons—solanine excluded—are altered into innocuousness by cooking; this is certainly not true of many of the additives. Third, the argument falls on its face when solanine is used as an example. My diary notes several cases of cures of long-standing depression when

61

potatoes and other members of the nightshade plants—including peppers, paprika, eggplant, and tomato—were removed from the diet. Not at all incidentally, these "natural poisons" are not without effects on other systems of the body. I have diary notes on a number of cases of osteoarthritis, ranging from mild to cripplingly severe, which were cured by abstention from nightshade plants. Originally, this was the research of a distinguished horticulturist, Dr. Norman F. Childers of Rutgers University. He demonstrated with thousands of subjects that one of the reactions to the nightshade plants in the diet may be—as it has been for grazing animals indiscreet enough to forage on them—crippling arthritis. His colleagues, many of them beneficiaries of a close tie with the agricultural industry, reacted to Childers' research by trying to prevent him from reading his papers at scientific meetings of horticultural researchers. The Arthritis Foundation, hopelessly wedded to hormone therapies, aspirin, and gold treatment for these diseases, called Childers' findings "at best, premature; at worst, false." One might reasonably think the same of the foundation's judgment. Please note, that this judgment, although it masquerades as fact, rests on a solid basis of no testing at all.

There are sometimes impacts on personality when development of a human being goes awry in the uterus or at puberty. One of these, the Morgagni Syndrome, is another example of physical disorders too frequently diagnosed as "all in the mind." It appears in short, hirsute, brunette women, usually obese, who show clear-cut symptoms of hypoglycemia but don't respond to any of the treatments for low blood sugar until, as Herman Goodman and I learned in years of wrestling with their symptoms, the hypoglycemia diet is supplemented with glycine, the simplest protein (amino) acid. The women suffer with fatigue, headache, sleepiness, lethargy, vertigo, and tinnitus (noises in the ears). The only physical abnormality correlated with this array of subjective symptoms is a thickening of the skull. Although glycine is manufactured in the body and is patently harmless, the FDA reacted to my publications on the subject by classifying it as a new drug. If the cat has kittens in the oven, you can call them biscuits, but the FDA's change in nomenclature required that glycine manufacturers spend millions of dollars to prove the worth of the amino acid. Since there are relatively few women with the Morgagni defect, the market doesn't warrant the effort and the money, and glycine disappeared from the shelves. Fortunately, I have found that whole gelatin is a rich enough source of the protein to serve the needs of these unfortunate women, and as yet the government has not changed *that* to a drug.

In the uterus begin the emotional-mental-physical problems of another and more numerous group of women, those who are cast on the scrap heap of medicine by being labeled "constitutionally inadequate." Their symptoms are calculated to catapult them onto the psychiatric couch, for they begin with a constant feeling of inadequacy in meeting responsibilities. Other symptoms are sensitivity of the skin to friction of tight-fitting or rough-textured garments, callusing of the feet, therapeutic dependence on coffee and cola drinks, because these people are always seeking a lift from fatigue, susceptibility to sore throats, with the pain frequently radiating up to the ears, bandlike headaches, and difficulty in expressing warmth, which in some of them is characterized by their husbands or lovers (may they never meet) as outright frigidity. The physical maldevelopment, which is the neglected clue to the origin of their problems, is the narrowness of their palate. The mouth is crowded—they are frequently compelled to seek orthodontic correction for their bite—and the middle third of the face, the part under the nose, is "pushed in," with the palate tending toward a Gothic arch rather than a broad curve. All this is counted as normal and certainly unrelated to their troubles. (For one thing, there are millions of people with narrow dental arches, and the average, remember, becomes the normal.) However, when we remember that the pituitary gland lies behind the palate and develops from the same tissue and at the same time in the embryo, it becomes obvious that interference with development of the upper mouth may similarly impede development of the pituitary gland. The thesis becomes more tenable when one feeds these women polyunsaturated fat, Vitamin E, PABA (para-amino-benzoic acid), Vitamin C, and such

63

trace minerals as copper, cobalt, manganese, and zinc, which are pituitary stimulants. Given the right doses—since overdose can drive the gland too much and actually intensify the symptoms—these women respond with a heightened sense of adequacy in facing their responsibilities and with mitigation or disappearance of many of the other symptoms. Premenstrual tension and the painful menstrual characteristic of many in this group are also relieved.

Years ago, when I gave a paper on this unrecognized syndrome at the New York Dental Society, a dentist asked what the corresponding syndrome is in men with narrow palates. When I answered that asocial behavior with particular emphasis on crimes of senseless violence may be the dominant effect, the dentist destroyed my thesis with a sweeping blow. "I have," he announced, "a number of male patients with narrow palates who never committed a crime." I agreed that there are many criminals with broad palates who nonetheless commit crimes of senseless violence, but if you think the practitioner's non sequitur discourages a nutritionist, you underestimate our conviction. We are still trying to persuade criminologists that there is a relationship between mind and body, and haven't even been discouraged by the letters we receive from convicts who are diabetic or hypoglycemic, or both, and can't persuade prison administrators that they need special diets. Nor can we convince them that attention to special nutritional needs might be money-saving, by shortening prison stay, and reducing recidivism. Oh, well—at how many windmills can one charge?

I was once lecturing and autographing books at a department store, which is part of the Inquisition which publishers inflict on authors. My lecture was on psychonutrition to which this chapter and one of my books are dedicated. A psychiatrist in the audience, obviously a faithful voice of the establishment in his field, had challenged some of my statements and encountered a storm of protest from those who from personal experience knew how mistaken he was. The last person on the long line waiting for their books to be autographed was a young woman, perhaps in her mid-twenties, who said something I shall never forget:

"I am a schizophrenic. I've been sick since I was thirteen years old, and I spent fifteen years in mental hospitals. I had shock therapy more times than I can remember, and all the drugs— even the experimental ones. Nothing helped me until I found your book. It gave me the strength and the will to try once again. With the help of my doctor, who didn't believe in you but wouldn't discourage me, I found my way back. I'm working by day—I took off to come here—and I go to school at night to catch up on the education I missed.

"I love you," she said, and was gone before I could respond.

Which answers a question I raised earlier: why would a man stay in a profession which with such facility stimulates allied health disciplines into sadism seasoned with contempt? Garnished with lethargy, resistance, and abuse from the very public he hopes to help? Because he sees you as captives of health technologies you neither control nor understand. Because he loves you. What other rational explanation could there be?

4

From MS to Strokes to Infertility

A group of physicians called me to invite me to a consultation in the case of a paralyzed young woman bedded in New York's Lenox Hill Hospital. I've been interested in nerve muscle disorders, or myoneuropathies in medical jargon, for the good reason that there is often help in my field where there is little in medicine. The doctors asked me to see the patient in the hope that I might be able to offer both a diagnosis and a treatment. Had I wanted to be a therapist, I'd have studied medicine or remained a clinical nutritionist, as I was early in my career, but the more I saw of treatment the more I realized that it did nothing but reaffirm the value of prevention.

I couldn't turn my back on a paralyzed girl, though, and with the three physicians, visited her in the hospital. I recognized the condition almost immediately, which didn't prove that I'm a great diagnostician, for I had seen it once before. I told the three physicians that the patient had brain damage, tentatively located the site, advised them that surgery probably wasn't feasible because only a few, inaccessible cells might be involved, and concluded by advising twenty-four-hour nursing care, because my experience with the previous patient indicated that there was a risk of episodes of asphyxiation. I also suggested a nutritional therapy, although I wasn't optimistic about the outcome.

As I walked down the long corridor toward the entrance, the doctors were behind me, and I heard one of them say, sotto voce: "That SOB is a Ph.D. and I treated him like an M.D.!" I couldn't resist telling him the story of the physician who returns home unexpectedly early and finds his wife in bed with another doctor. Outraged, he yanks her out of the extramarital bed, screaming, "Are you aware that that man is not a member of the AMA?"

At the time of this incident I was having a battle with my own family physician, and I was stirred into writing this letter to him:

"Dear Doctor: I have learned not to complain when my urgent call finds you playing golf or driving in your new sports car, for which I'm sure I paid. I submit without protest to serving as a new slate on which your inexperienced assistant can practice his prescription writing. And I no longer debate when you insist that you can't practice competent medicine in the home, with the result that I must take my feverish, dehydrated, and nauseated child to the hospital emergency room to keep a medical tryst with you.

"But I can't keep silent when you cure with magic names. I came to you with a backache, and after excluding numerous unnamed diseases which occur twice a year in two subjects in Africa, you triumphantly announced that I had lumbago, which would automatically have made me feel better if I didn't know that it means backache. Then you wrote a prescription for an eight-syllable something-or-other which turned out to be aspirin combined with an antacid, at three times the price of Bufferin. Aside from making me $39.90 poorer, all that you accomplished was to motivate me into going to a chiropractor who showed me something you missed on the X ray, and then proceeded to cure me. He's a quack, of course, by your definition, but I notice that some of your peers in medicine have formed a society of 'manipulative medicine,' which obviously translates as: if you can't lick 'em, join them in chiropractic by another name.

"Speaking of your attitude toward 'inferior' professions: it also sticks in my throat every time I read an article written by a physician for laymen, because somewhere in it will be a phrase the typesetters must keep permanently set for medical writing. It goes: "Only your physician is qualified to" whatever it is: diagnose, maldiagnose, prescribe, treat—or overlook? What is the basic insecurity in your profession that makes it necessary for you to reassure yourselves in this way? The same anxiety is reflected in your code of ethics. You may consult with other professions, but you must not treat them as equals unless their training is identical with yours. Ever thought of flouting the code by treating other professions as *superior?* The herbalist, the osteopath, the chiropractor, and, yes, the nutritionist all have something to offer, and usually it's distinctly *not* based on training identical with yours.

"I am profoundly disturbed, too, by your apparent belief that for each symptom, if not for each ailment, there is, or there will one day be, a wonder drug—the wonder being, I suppose, that the patient survives the side reactions. We already have a happy pill for depression, a calmer for euphoria, a sedative for sleep and a stimulant to offset it, a hormone for arthritis, and another to allow malnourished, infertile women to become malnourished, fertile mothers of unhealthy babies. It is apparent that most of this witch's brew is used for symptomatic relief, which represents a type of medicine you surely were trained to avoid. How will you be viewed a century from now? And with what hostility will your profession regard the biochemists, enzymologists, and nutritionists as they take over medicine, which they will?

"Much of what I have just written was inspired by our last conversation, when I tried to help you in the management of your brother's multiple sclerosis. When I suggested to you that a nutritional treatment which I've tested on more than 300 patients over a period of a quarter of a century was, though no panacea, harmless and well worth testing for your brother, you didn't even ask me for a description of the diet and the supplements. Afraid your fellow physicians might consider you a food faddist? We could have kept the whole disgraceful episode a dark secret, even if your brother improved. Nutritionists aren't bound by the medical ethic concerning privileged communication, but we do observe it.

"Instead of investigating what I was telling you, you remarked, in a tone implying that only a physician could possibly know, that multiple sclerosis patients have a tendency to spontaneous recoveries, with or without treatment, so that any concomitant treatment is given credit. That neatly disposed of my successful cases. I wasn't about to tell you the dark secret: nutritionists are aware of spontaneous recoveries in multiple sclerosis, and I have developed a technique which at least in some patients will identify an induced (rather than fortuitous) recovery. So your brother will continue to lose ground, and you will remain respectable. All this despite the fact that I can give you the names of a dozen physicians who have used my therapy successfully.

"Before I end this diatribe, I must do something about your complacency, and I should be able to do that by asking you if the demyelination* of the nerve sheaths in multiple sclerosis is permanent. If you are honest, you will acknowledge that it *is*. And if it is, how do you explain the spontaneous recoveries? Sincerely."

I'll confess that my doctor caught a tide of indignation for which his immobile complacency was not solely responsible. At the time, I had had a brush with the multiple sclerosis society in my home area and I was still seething. That story can be pieced together from the following notes in my diary.

The father of a young man with multiple sclerosis called me at the suggestion of his physician. I agreed to supply the data concerning the nutritional therapy to the doctor, but the caller asked me to delay for a month. He had been advised to take his son, who was in a wheelchair, to Liberty, New York, to try a cold climate for him. I couldn't resist remarking that MS patients have a very low resistance to stress, and cold weather for them is a great stress. But the father was committed to the journey and promised to call me on his return, which he did. The patient had appreciably worsened in the cold climate, as might have been anticipated—even a tooth extraction can set these patients back significantly. Now at the father's request, the doctor called, seeking details of the therapy which I supplied. Three months later the father called again, jubilantly reporting that his son had

*Loss of the insulation which keeps nerves from "short-circuiting."

regained the ability to hold his head upright, to exercise bladder and bowel control, to control his eyes, and to speak coherently. I had suggested a handwriting comparison at the beginning and at the end of the treatment, for writing is a skilled neurological feat, and progress with it can be used to distinguish between spontaneous and induced recovery. The young man held his improvement for nearly a year (perhaps longer, for I didn't get a report from the doctor) when the father called again. He wanted to know if the multiple sclerosis society was aware of the nutritional treatment. I said that I had sent them details in response to their inquiries several times, with no response. The father grimly remarked that he had contributed thousands of dollars to the society, and he would see to it that what I was espousing received an objective investigation and a clinical trial.

A month later, a medical man with the society called and asked for the data concerning the therapy and the names of physicians who had applied it. I supplied the information. Months of silence followed. I called the physicians, a dozen of them, whose names I had given to the medical man, and learned that none of them had heard from him. I then wrote to the society, under an assumed name, saying that I was an MS patient and interested in Dr. Fredericks' nutritional therapy. What could they tell me about it? There came the immortal answer, which I quote verbatim: "Dr. Fredericks' therapy is valueless, and we have never tested it."

Well, it has been said that large institutions tend to preserve the status quo—which is the mess we're in.

At intervals the society has again queried me, but I have not replied. I don't want to give them the task of not testing the treatment again. But I have sent the information to hundreds of physicians all over the world sometimes getting very unexpected comments. I'm thinking of a Boston physician who wrote to me concerning a patient totally crippled with MS and confessed that he was hostile to the concept of nutritional treatment for the disorder and wrote only at his patient's insistence. I again supplied the data and, as I always do, asked for a progress report. It arrived six months or so later and, believe it or not, the letter read:

"Now that my patient is walking, can I stop the treatment?"

Talk about a left-handed report! My diary reminds me of another, a classic of its kind. I was in New Orleans lecturing at a convention. (Adelle Davis was there and called me at an early hour to invite me to have breakfast with her. I accepted, and she said, "I hope you don't mind my calling you at seven in the morning." To which I gallantly responded: "I'd rather you nudged me." There was a moment of silence, then Adelle replied, "Carlton, you made my whole day!")

Several years later I flew to Jacksonville, Florida, where I was met at the airport by the owner of a local health food store. As we drove toward town, he asked if I remembered talking to him at the New Orleans convention. I apologized, making my usual remark about the thousands of people I meet, whereupon he brought the car to a stop and very deliberately pulled his trousers up high enough to expose his knees. Before I had time to ask the significance of this male striptease, he said, "No braces!" He explained that at New Orleans he had asked me about the nutritional treatment for multiple sclerosis and brought me to his physician, who was also attending the convention, to outline the therapy, which I did.

"At the time," he said, "I was wearing braces on both legs— I had been medically discharged from the army because of the MS. You may have cost me my disability pension," he grinned, "and you don't even remember talking to me. I'll never forget it—not only because it helped me, but because everything you wanted my doctor to give me was on the shelves of my own health food store staring me in the face while I shuffled around on braces for four years. *That's* unforgettable."

He went on to tell me that his recovery had sparked a long-dormant ambition. He was going back to college to take a Ph.D., and for his thesis he proposed an investigation into nutrition in multiple sclerosis. He sold two of his stores, left his wife in charge of a third, and launched his doctoral candidacy with high hopes— which I didn't share. I knew he'd need the supervision of a medical man with experience in the management of MS, which would automatically alert the medical establishment to the pres-

71

ence of an interloper on the medical scene. So it proved. My friend's medical collaborator suddenly found it impossible to spare time for the project, and solicitation of others proved fruitless. He dropped his candidacy and is back in the health food business. He's still navigating splendidly without his leg braces, and still selling the "faddist" foods and supplements which helped him to become once more a whole man.

Since these are case histories with no double-blind devices to "control" the study, orthodox science will reject them out of hand, insisting that I am observing a "placebo" effect—the effect of the power of suggestion. Anything is possible, of course, but the first case of MS for which I was a consultant came in 1952. The man was badly crippled with the disease and he is still working (for Amtrak), handling heavy freight, twenty-seven years later. *That's* a mighty potent power of suggestion!

Because I've mentioned numerous consultations with physicians, don't assume that my relationship with medical men has been a long honeymoon. I remember without consulting my diary an aggravated example of the suspicion with which some physicians, stalwarts of the establishment, view nutritionists. I was testifying at a congressional hearing when I suddenly found myself under personal attack by one Tim Lee Carter, M.D., a congressman from Kentucky. Among other choice tidbits, he made the statement—before the wire services and television cameras—that I was falsely claiming a Ph.D. degree which, he said, I never acquired. After the National Health Federation pressured him into calling New York University and verifying my "imaginary" degree, he apologized—in public, but without the reporters and TV cameras. The accusation reached the media, but the apology and retraction did not.

I subsequently wrote to the congressman, inviting him to lunch on the basis that by then he must have realized that he had been supplied with misinformation—not only concerning me but concerning the bill we were discussing, which was aimed at stopping the FDA from inflicting a prescription requirement on vitamin supplements. He never replied, and for once I lost my temper and wrote a note to Dr. Carter which, among other remarks, suggested:

"You came to the hearing to meet the charlatan from New York. I came to meet the gentleman from Kentucky. How sad that we were both disappointed!"

My diary carries a memo on another note, addressed to President Richard M. Nixon's staff and written when I was the target of a determined effort by the FDA to silence my criticisms of that agency. The President had had inquiries made to learn if I would be interested in a "high federal position" which was not described. By the grapevine, I learned that this was the commissionership of the FDA. Knowing that no consumer-oriented commissioner would survive the lobbying of the medical political action committees, I told the President: "I'm not interested in the position you have in mind, but should you ever appoint an agency to protect the public against the FDA, I'll be glad to serve on it." I never heard from him again.

Many other memories come up with any mention of octocosanol as a neuromuscular factor. In addition to Bonnie, whose history you read about in the introduction to this book, and the many multiple sclerosis patients who have benefited from therapy with this wheat-germ oil concentrate, I include my mother, who was the victim of a stroke which had left her with one-sided paralysis and difficulties in speech. I told her physician that I would adminster octocosanol plus bioflavonoids and Vitamin C, a regimen calculated to strengthen the smaller blood vessels which, contrary to popular legend, are often the site of the "blow-out" which underlies a cerebral accident. Mother made an uneventful and complete recovery. Observing this unexpected event, the doctor then applied the treatment in a dozen cases of stroke with gratifying results for the entire group. His final comment was illuminating. "There are spontaneous recoveries in strokes," he warned, "—but don't stop what you're doing!" How does one establish the thin line behind scientific skepticism and unscientific cynicism?

My diary records my musings as I tried to explain the mechanism by which octocosanol helped brain-injured patients. There were three possibilities: (1) The concentrate stimulated the maturation of young nerve cells (neuroblasts) until they were able to take over the function of the damaged area. (2) The concentrate

73

actually stimulated repair of the damaged nerve cells. (3) The concentrate stimulated the brain into "rewiring" around the damaged area. Theory number 2, I felt, could be discarded. My neurology professor, like all neurology professors and textbooks, insisted that damaged nerves in the brain can't be repaired.

I took my questions to Dr. Andrew Ivy, a great physiologist. I told him the responses of the patients were sometimes too fast to allow for repair of damaged nerves, if that were possible, and too fast for stimulation of maturation of young nerve cells. Therefore the only tenable theory would be rewiring of brain circuits, which conceivably might be quickly achieved. Dr. Ivy silenced me with a single statement. "You're repairing damaged cerebral neurons (cells)," he said. "I know you were taught this is impossible—but the textbooks are wrong. I have unpublished work in my own lab to prove that." Which left me nowhere, for one can't cite unpublished research to buttress a theory, and observation of repair is almost impossible to achieve. But that is really the only tenable explanation of some of the dividends from administration of this wheat-germ oil concentrate in epilepsy of traumatic origin, in minimal brain damage, in MS, and in strokes.

Which brings us to the old question, the asking of which is the hallmark of the food faddist: why do they take the wheat germ out of flour? Answer: no self-respecting weevil, mold, or fungus, unless in desperation, will try to feed on food which will not support life. Which brings up the outraged reaction of the FDA when I broadcast the news that the proposed standards for white bread, called to my attention by Senator Paul Douglas, would make *illegal* an improved loaf such as the Cornell formula, which is higher in protein, vitamins, and minerals and rich in wheat germ. This brought thousands of letters to the federal agency, which responded with a release dutifully carried in *The New York Times*: "Food Faddists Show Strong Hold on Public."

The subject of wheat-germ oil brings back memories of its mistaken identification as a source of nothing more than Vitamin E, and the subsequent misidentification of Vitamin E as the middle letter in the word *sex*. I tried to straighten out that misconcept in many broadcasts, in the course of which—as in some of my books—I devoted considerable effort to nutritional improvement of fertility. It is an illusion, created by the millions spent in advertising paper diapers, that our population is sexually and reproductively efficient. The fact is that about an estimated 10 percent of our marriages are involuntarily barren. Why else would there be a black market in adoption of babies? Add to that the sizable percentage of pregnancies which do not produce a live, healthy baby and the percentage which yield malformed or retarded children, and you have a reproductive record which in a stable for thoroughbred horses would be regarded as a disaster.

In response to one of these broadcasts, a young woman appeared at the studio asking for help in achieving motherhood. A consulting physician indicated that she had a tilted uterus, and although thousands of babies have spilled out of tilted uteruses, she dutifully submitted to surgical correction. Her husband had a low sperm count, and was placed on improved nutrition, which she shared. After six months she appeared again at the broadcast, indicated her impatience, and asked what could be done to speed the process. I protested that she had been wrestling with her problem for years and was giving good nutrition only a few months, but my comments made no impression. I finally suggested artificial insemination, explaining that her husband's sperm would be mixed with the sperm of a donor who would physically resemble her husband and be in excellent health. She rushed out of the studio, returned with her bashful husband in tow and a determined look in her eye, and said to my secretary, "We decided we'd like our child to be a nutritionist." My secretary explained that I was at stud only in alternate years. (P.S. The woman had her baby, and promptly achieved another successful pregnancy. My diary doesn't record it, but I don't understand women.)

5
Tilting at the Establishment Windmills

My older son was working as a technician in a hospital operating room when a surgeon discovered his identity and remarked, "I disagree with everything in your father's books. Who wrote them for him?" My son, from whom I always say I inherited my quick wit, answered, "Who read them to you?" He lost his job. But he said it was worth it.

Surgeons, like all medical men, resent flak from those they call "paraprofessionals." I'm not sure that nonmedical nutritionists have as yet been promoted to that level, but the surgeons in any case have been resistant to our pleas that patients destined for elective surgery should be prepared nutritionally. This certainly doesn't mean the usual preoperative starvation, garnished with intravenous glucose (sugar). And emergency surgery doesn't justify the sugar diet either, in lieu of the stress-resisting nutrients needed in generous amounts to meet the heightened requirements of a sick person about to encounter the insults of anesthesia and surgery. So it has been that those of us in nutrition can add the surgeons to the long list of medical specialists who hold that the diet of the hospitalized patient is the province of the dietitian, however enamored she may be—and they often are—of overcooked vegetables, emasculated white bread, salads of anemic tomato and discouraged lettuce, and such desserts as Jell-O, which is 85 percent sugar and gleams with coal-tar dyes.

That paragraph gives you a short perspective on one source of hostility toward nutritionists. Add that of the food processors, the Better Business Bureaus which think food processors need protection from the public, the trade associations, the captive professors who eat industry bread and sing its song, the dietitians who reject any concept not embalmed in their outdated textbooks, the newspaper food columnists who don't step on the toes of food advertisers, and the government agencies subservient to the pressures of agribusiness—and you can understand that an honest, competent, objective nutritionist might regard India's Untouchables as a privileged class.

When the case of the hostile is weak, it is classical, if an admission of intellectual bankruptcy, to attack the man rather than the issue. So it has been, more frequently in bygone years, that I've found my training described as being in physical education, recreation, journalism, or communications. That always amuses me, because whenever I feel like exercising I summon my willpower and lie down until the feeling departs. Recreation is something the public gave me no time for, and it would seem reasonable that my forty-odd years as an author, newspaper columnist, radio and TV broadcaster, and teacher would be a satisfactory substitute for academic classroom theories of mass communications. Actually, just to keep the record straight, my earned graduate degrees are both in public health education, and my doctoral dissertation was a study of the effectiveness of mass education in nutrition—the field in which I've specialized for four decades. Nonetheless, I've been brought under fire because, my critics point out, my university curricula included no courses labeled "nutrition." They carefully omit the fact that I didn't take such courses because I was asked to teach them—at some half-dozen colleges and universities, ranging from the dental school of U.C.L.A. to N.Y.U. and Fairleigh Dickinson. Moreover, nutrition was a segment of many of my courses, which is the same way many physicians received their nutrition education. I also paralleled the medical men when I studied nutrition in some 200 hours of continuing medical education courses. Nonetheless, if you write to the FDA concerning my background, you will find me described, depending on what file they draw on, as a journalist, as the holder of a Ph.D. in recreation, as a self-styled nutritionist, ad infinitum, ad nauseam. May I suggest that a Ph.D. and Phi Beta Kappa single-mindedly concentrating on a single field for four decades might be considered to have accumulated *some* valid information.

My thirty-year battle with the FDA will become understandable when I tell you the story of a little girl whose pediatrician consulted me because he wasn't happy about her progress. Her problem was osteomyelitis, a chronic bone infection for which there is a chronic (and obviously unsuccessful) treatment consisting of removal of dying bone and doses of penicillin. I suggested to the pediatrician the use of nutritional support in the form of cod-liver oil, large doses of Vitamin C, and a small amount of calcium orotate, a form of the mineral which is better utilized than the more commonly used calcium preparations. The pediatrician reported a few months later that Susie was for the first time being permitted full activity in school. The lesions had healed and, he said, "You have our orthopedist looking at the X rays, shaking his head, and muttering 'Impossible!' " The case will never be recorded in the annals of medicine, not only because it's a single history, but because we didn't have a second Susie with osteomyelitis of the ankle, pelvis, and skull, treated with "spurious" vitamins and "imitation" minerals, to rule out the power of suggestion. I put it to you solemnly that there never has been a case of osteomyelitis that yielded to faith healing, and in any case, Susie had no faith in me—I was the consultant who made her parents deny her the pleasures of junk food.

The other point to this story is the history of calcium orotate. Although calcium and orotic acid, from which this compound is made, are normal to the body, the FDA decided to label this harmless supplement a "new drug," which will make it unobtainable until someone spends a million to comply with the "new drug regulations." No one will, however, because the product can't be patented and the money will have been spent to make competitive marketers of the product rich. So the memory of Susie is clouded by the realization that other sufferers will not receive the possible benefits of the nutritional treatment because a simple (and more effective) calcium supplement, thanks to bureaucratic fiat, will not be available.

Even as I wrote those lines I received a call from a Cornell nutritionist asking me for data he needs to oppose new FDA regulations which have been proposed for the manufacture and sale of vitamin supplements. One of their proposals is to ban marketing of para-amino-benzoic acid (PABA), a vitamin which has kept me personally twenty years younger than my age, and to place Vitamin E on a list of substances not generally regarded as safe. What is fascinating about the Vitamin E ruling will not be readily apparent until I tell you that it is a harmless substitute for estrogen in the treatment of menopausal flushes, while estrogen, which is known to cause cancer, will still be readily available.* And you have just read the type of statement which embroiled me in a battle with the FDA over a period of more than a quarter of a century, during which the agency deviated into a sensible approach to vitamins on only one occasion that I can remember: when they decided to say nothing.

In the middle of my candidacy for the Ph.D. in public health education, the battle with the FDA via radio, TV, and my newspaper columns was at its height. Inspired by the resentful government agency, a group of physicians called N.Y.U. to announce that in their opinion and that of the U.S. government I was not a suitable candidate for a doctoral degree. The dean asked me to offset the telephone campaign by requesting my medical friends to write to him endorsing my competence and character, as he believed with obvious logic that letters would carry more weight than telephone calls. Among the physicians I called was a gynecologist I had met some years before when the circulation in his legs was so poor that he was threatened with bilateral amputation. He came to my office to explore what

*This was the specific advice given to a physician who queried the *JAMA*, seeking a substitute for estrogen in the treatment of a woman whose history of breast cancer made the hormone therapy too risky!

nutrition had to offer, and ten years later danced at my wedding on the legs he was supposed to have lost. Nonetheless, the grateful physician refused to write an endorsing letter to the university. "It wouldn't," he explained with great sincerity, "be ethical."

While official medicine was doing its best to impugn my competence, members of the profession not infrequently called upon me for help. One such inquiry came from the head of the myasthenia gravis clinic of a major New York hospital. Myasthenia gravis is the threatening disorder of the muscles which, if you remember, was one of the terminal problems of Aristotle Onassis, who found it necessary to tape his eyelids to keep them from closing. Treatment of this lethal disorder, which I believe sometimes to be triggered by intolerance to potato, tomato, and other plants of the nightshade family, ordinarily consists of doses of drugs which stimulate production in the body of acetylcholine, a neurotransmitter which makes possible communication between the nervous systems and the muscles. Lack of that neurotransmitter in the brain can be responsible for memory defects and for a type of senility, a chemistry based on nutrition once called "food faddism" by the establishment and now official doctrine thanks to Wurtman's research at M.I.T. The drug treatment for myasthenia gravis fails sometimes because the patient becomes resistant to the drugs or because he becomes *too* responsive. What follows then (a cholinergic crisis, they call it) may end in death, as the disease process, unchecked, often does. The myasthenia gravis specialist had a patient who had stopped responding to medication, could no longer chew or swallow, and was losing weight at an alarming rate. His query: "Could you provide an adequate liquid diet which would halt the weight loss, and perhaps reverse it?"

I suggested that nutrition offered more in myasthenia gravis than a good liquid diet—that it might be possible nutritionally to offset some of the defect in acetylcholine synthesis, thereby anticipating by twenty years M.I.T.'s triumphant "breakthrough." I reminded the physician that acetylcholine originates with nutritional factors—as, indeed, do all the body's chemicals.

Whence else? Following the nutritional therapy—doses of manganese, choline, and pantothenic acid—the patient regained some of her muscle tone, began to chew and swallow normally, and gained twelve pounds in four weeks. A newspaper reporter, a woman who made a living by attacking all avant-garde nutritionists, including me, heard a rumor about the case and interviewed the doctor. He severely criticized the claims which the reporter said I'd made (although I actually had said nothing about the case to her or anyone else), and remarked: "The recovery of the patient was entirely due to the delayed effect of our previous treatment." I can assure you that, had she died, it most certainly would not have been a "delayed effect of her previous treatment." And had the doctor granted that her journey toward death was really slowed, if not interrupted, by the nutritional therapy, myasthenia gravis patients would today be receiving harmless nutritional treatments, minus the threat of the "cholinergic crisis." But it would have required every inch of the physician's stature as an authority to try, alone, to reverse medical apathy toward nutrition. It wasn't apathy, in those days, but hostility—we tend to be down on what we're not up on.

That attitude, incidentally, isn't confined to the medical profession, as I learned in an encounter with a veterinarian who was treating our little schnauzer, who had barely survived an argument with a speeding car. Scruffy had numerous fractures, three in one small leg, several in his ribs, and the ligament at the hip area of the fractured leg was so torn that it looked like crumpled cellophane in the X ray. Were the schnauzer not the Frederickses' dog, said the vet, he would have put him to sleep. Reluctantly he applied casts—several of which Scruffy promptly chewed off—and warned that the animal would drag that leg for the rest of his life, and that a fenced run must be provided for him, since he would not be able to defend himself against other dogs.

I told the vet that I would give Scruffy high-quality protein, particularly eggs, and supplements of Vitamin C, Vitamin E, calcium, magnesium, and wheat-germ oil. He challenged only the Vitamin C. Dogs make their own, he said. But who could

assure us that Scruffy, under stress, would raise his internal synthesis of Vitamin C to the high level needed to accelerate healing?

Four weeks later Scruffy was navigating on all four legs. I
pointed out to the veterinarian that the serial X rays showed
complete restoration of the "permanently destroyed ligament" as
well as the fractures, and urged him to write a paper on the case.
"Not me," said the animal doctor. "I'm a devout coward—I have
no desire to be the Carlton Fredericks of the veterinarians."

These minor skirmishes behind the scenes occasionally erupted
in full view of the public. A striking example of the establishment
in full flight from a new idea came when I accepted an invitation
from the Huxley Institute to lecture for their Washington chapter,
which had secured a permit to use an auditorium in the National
Institutes of Health building. With obvious malice, the permit
for the use of the auditorium in the government building was
withdrawn a few hours before the event, leaving the Huxley group
to face irate ticketholders who were coming to Washington for
the event from some ten or eleven states. There was no way to
advise the audience of the cancellation. The excuse was that the
NIH require that the member who sponsors a meeting has to be
an expert in the field reflected in the lecture, which in this case
was orthomolecular psychiatry, as an improvement on the couch,
conversation, calmative drugs, and shock therapy. Our sponsor
had no such qualifications; indeed, it was entirely possible that
no one associated with NIH could claim such expertise.

We instigated indignant calls of protest from several dozen
congressmen and senators, but their objections were met with
stalling tactics, although we did establish the fact that no previous
meeting had ever before been canceled on such grounds.

I was as determined as the Huxley Institute group that the
public should hear the lecture, and joined forces with Marlene
David of the Federal Trade Commission and Clinton Miller of
the National Health Federation in a search for another auditorium which could seat at least 500. We located a room in a
Holiday Inn across the street from the giant NIH building, which
we circled with pickets to intercept the audience, since we didn't
know what entrances they might use. And we succeeded in stag-

ing the lecture. In fact, we succeeded four times, because the room only held 150, and I had to repeat my talk until everyone who desired to had the opportunity to hear it. I reached my bed at 2:00 A.M., exhausted but satisfied. The shabbiness of the tactics of the NIH hierarchy only increased my determination to encourage the psychotic, the neurotic, the autistic, the depressed, and the senile to escape from the clutches of orthodox psychiatry, which I predict will, like psychoanalysis, the Zeppelin, the dinosaur, the auk, and the dodo, one day be regarded as a singular event of a primitive era.

While I'm on the topic of psychiatry, let me pause to tell you a family story involving the profession, one I've never been able to sneak by the reticences of TV and radio. We Frederickses have a remarkable granddaughter—doesn't everyone?—whose father, a physician, took her to the golf course, thereby combining babysitting with another favorite pastime. Morgan, three years old, joined her father in the locker room, and was fascinated by her first encounter with a number of naked adult males. Pointing a small finger, she asked: "What's *that*?" Her father reacted with his normal medical terminology: "That's a penis," he said. Asked Morgan: "Do I have one?" Told she did not, she asked: "Does mother have one?" Told she also did not, she said to her father: "But *you* have one." When her father agreed, Morgan hastened to reassure him. "Don't worry about it," she urged. "It's very small." A nearby psychiatrist, overhearing the conversation, allowed that Freud had spoken only of penis envy—not pity.

Alcoholism is a problem obviously involving chemistries unique to alcoholics. Despite that patent fact, the psychiatric establishment desperately resists nutritional approaches to the problems of addicts, just as it resists the concept that there is more than one type of alcoholism. It's obvious that we in nutrition can't communicate with those who insist that psychotherapy, Antabuse, shock treatment, and concessions to a Higher Power are the sole answers to "the" problem. In chapter 1, I shared with you a letter from a male addict who conquered his appetite for alcohol when he adopted the hypoglycemia diet. This labels him as a hypoglycemic who became a drinker, which is to say that the first disorder triggered the second. But when you discuss this with the establishment in the field, they reply that *all* alcoholics become hypoglycemic, for the blood sugar must drop when they substitute whiskey for food. The psychiatrist seems to have a blind spot which keeps him from realizing that the hypoglycemia may come first and initiate the drinking, these sufferers substituting alcohol for the sweets usually craved by those with low blood sugar. But then, they are also light-years away from recognizing that there are at least two other types of addiction, one based on allergy and another on inordinately high requirements for certain nutrients.

The journey from hypoglycemia into alcoholism was once described for my wife by a former showgirl whom she met in a dress shop. Identifying Betty as my wife, she said that she owed me a letter of gratitude, and asked her to repeat to me the story she told. She had had no troubles until she had her baby. "Then," she said, "I became more and more tired and nervous, and I discovered that a drink in the morning helped me to face the day. That progressed into all-day drinking, with bottles hidden all over the house. By that time, I was desperate. My husband wouldn't have been sympathetic, so I went to a psychiatrist three times a week. That didn't help. I was lying in bed one morning, too weak to get up and shut off the radio, which my little boy had turned on, and I became a captive audience for Dr. Fredericks as he discussed a type of alcoholism which, he said, could be started by low blood sugar. My predrinking symptoms matched his list for hypoglycemia, so I asked my doctor to test me for it. He refused, and so did the psychiatrist. I told the two of them I'd find a new doctor, and they surrendered, ordered the test, and said the results were 'borderline.'

"By that time, though, I had your husband's book, and I'd learned enough from it to realize that 'borderline' results should not be ignored but treated, so I went on the diet anyway. A few weeks later, I found I could take or leave a drink, and sometime later I lost the desire."

Betty faithfully carried the message to me, and I added it to the case histories with which I tried to persuade the establishment in alcoholism to take a fresh view of the problem. I added the comments made by the founder of AA, who was very much impressed by the responses of alcoholics to orthomolecular (nutritional) treatment; and I accomplished nothing. Predictably, I was repeatedly assured that low blood sugar is not a cause but a *result* of alcoholism. I *know* they're wrong. I also know what the Scriptures mean when they describe a eunuch, lying on a woman and groaning heavily.

That same feeling of frustration engulfs me when I hear, as I have often, a young medical man say that geriatrics—the care of the aged—offers no challenges. What can you accomplish? In response, there are three stories I tell, one of which concerns the lawyer in the old age home you have already read about in chapter 2. Let me add two others. For many years I was the beneficiary of the medical knowledge of Dr. Herman Goodman, who co-authored one of my books. He asked me to accompany him to the home of an eighty-four-year-old woman who was, he said, in terminal coma—dying of no particular disease but disintegrating like the one-horse shay. He was about to start procaine therapy, which you would recognize if I called it Novocaine, the familiar local anesthetic your dentist uses. In nutrition we recognize procaine as a source of an anti-aging factor, PABA or para-amino-benzoic acid, supplements of which have long retarded graying of my hair and helped me to retain the characteristics of youth which, my wife vows, could only have been achieved by a pact with the devil.

When we got to the woman's house, Dr. Goodman administered 5 cc's of the procaine by intramuscular injection, accompanied by a second injection of Vitamin B Complex. He continued this treatment for several months, and then one day invited me to see the patient again. When we got to the house, the maid met us at the door and invited us to come in and wait. "Madame," she told us, "is taking her morning walk in the park."

The incident is indelibly registered in my memory, for years later I had the opportunity to recommend similar treatment to another physician also struggling with a failing patient deep in her eighties. He too asked me to join him in his house call, also remarking that the patient was dying of no particular disease. In fact, he said, he didn't know what he would put on the death certificate. After seeing the patient, I suggested rectal feeding with glucose (medicine then didn't have the "hyperalimentation" liquids of today, which are given intravenously) accompanied by 15-cc injections of Vitamin B Complex. (It's a grievous error to give sugar without the B vitamins; you simply intensify the already serious vitamin deficiencies of an aged patient. But only nutritionists know this, and we've obviously kept it a secret.) The "normal" dose of injectable Vitamin B Complex was, at most, 2 cc's. The doctor gulped, but gamely complied with the regimen, returning every day to renew the treatment. Months passed, and he called me again. "I'm going to see the patient—you remember her?" I didn't—there had been too many consultations, too many notes in the diary in those months. We rang the bell at the modest Brooklyn brownstone house, but no one responded, and finding the door open, we entered. From the "parlor," a forgotten term of a long-ago Brooklyn (but then, the portiere was, if you please, made of varicolored glass beads, and the lamps were original Tiffany), came the sound of typing. There sat a little old lady, a shawl around her shoulders, typing at a mad rate. Over her shoulder she said, "Excuse me, Doctor, I left the door open for you, because I have to finish my script. I'm on television tomorrow to show my handicrafts, and for me, you know, it's always later than you think."

Glucose and the Vitamin B Complex are no panaceas for the malnourished elderly. The important point is that this woman lived and *functioned* for years, a span and privilege that would have been denied if the physician had leaned only on the drugs of allopathic medicine. When I have told this and similar stories in past years, medical men have recoiled; one could almost hear the term *faddism* trembling on their lips. Today, there are "hyperalimentation" committees in most hospitals. The term is medicalese for concentrated superfeeding. It's done in emergencies, as usual. But in the inevitable course of events it may occur to a pioneering physician, someday, that supernutrition can be applied *before* the crisis—by mouth, not by vein, and at home, not in the hospital. Matters may even develop to the point that medicine will realize that the elderly in the outpatient clinics are (a) candidates for later hospital stays, (b) malnourished right now, and (c) less likely to be hospitalized, or better candidates for therapy, if preventive nutrition is applied before the crisis demands feeding by vein.

Years ago, when I had time to speak at service clubs, such as Rotary, Lion, or Kiwanis (where they feed you terrible food and then sit back to hear a lecture on good nutrition), I encountered a physician who seemed very interested in my remarks on the dividends from nutritional preparation for surgery. I met him again, twenty-five years later, as I approached my classroom at a university. Nutritionists not being allowed to age—indeed, to die, unless we're hit by a UFO—he recognized me, and we chatted for a few minutes. "I'm a surgeon," he said, "and since that talk at the Rotary Club, I made it a point whenever not in the grip of a surgical emergency to prepare my patients for operations with well-balanced meals, supplements of protein, and high doses of vitamins and minerals. And I can tell you that my records show a very satisfying drop in complications and deaths ever since."

I wanted to know if he had shared his secret with other surgeons. He said it was wonderful that after all these years of battling, I managed to remain naive and hopeful.

6

Help for Women, and Men, and Both

April, our four-year old, was supposed to be waiting in the hotel lobby while Betty dressed, but when my wife came down there was no April, and a half-hour search of the lobby, its shops, and the nearby Miami Beach neighborhood didn't turn up our beautiful little daughter. As Betty went from panic to hysteria and was about to call the police, two six-footers, black-suited and white-tied, entered the lobby, one of them bearing April astride his massive shoulders. Moreover, she wasn't wearing the clothing with which she'd left the room, but was exquisitely dressed in a costly hand-dyed skirt and blouse, with shoes and socks to match. When Betty identified herself as April's mother, the men explained that April had wandered by them as they were studying the racing charts. Having had a very bad day in their choices of horses, they asked the child to make a selection. She placed her innocent finger on a long shot which promptly won the race, paying $22. They celebrated their bonanza by taking April to an exclusive children's shop for a new wardrobe.

When they established Betty's identity as my wife they were delighted, for both, they announced, were faithful listeners to my broadcasts. Learning that I was in New York, they appointed themselves as bodyguards for my family. The following night, a young man attempted to strike up a conversation with Betty in the dining room. His intentions may have been pristine pure, but the two horseplayers appeared as if dropped from the ceiling and carried him out of the dining room between them, his feet not touching the floor. As they left with their terrified captive, one of them shook a massive fist in the offender's face and warned him: "And anudda t'ing! Mudderhood is sacrid!" Damon Runyon would have had a sense of nostalgia.

However sacred motherhood is, our medical culture certainly doesn't pull out the stops in trying to help the millions of married couples who can't conceive children. It's estimated that at least 10 percent of our marriages are involuntarily barren, and though veterinarians put a high priority on correct nutrition for animal reproductive efficiency, it is the thought after the last resort of the specialists in human infertility. When I went before a medical society devoted to the subject to give a paper on nutrition in reproduction, I was told I was the only speaker on that subject in the twenty-year history of the organization. I thought at that moment of the primitive peoples who insist that married couples defer conception until both of them are nutritionally prepared. I thought of the Maori mother-in-law, who walks endless miles to the sea so that her daughter-in-law's pregnancy diet may contain enough fish. I thought of the South Seas ethnic group who reproach mothers who have had a miscarriage or a defective baby, remarking, "You have only yourself to blame—you didn't eat properly." And I thought also of an obstetrician's response to a nauseated pregnant woman worried about the inadequacy of her diet: "That baby is only the size of a fist," he told her. "Its nutritional needs are so minute that there's nothing to worry about." That flying flag of opinionated ignorance dismayed me, knowing that the matrixes—the blueprints—for all the baby's organs are laid down in the first few months. That's why thalidomide caused such havoc when prescribed early in pregnancy but was innocuous when taken much later.

I bring this matter up for reasons beyond the importance of nutrition in maintaining reproductive efficiency. There is good reason to believe that Vitamin B_6 deficiency, rather than an oversupply of cholesterol, may be the prime cause of pathological hardening of the arteries. Cholesterol *can't* be responsible for that condition when early signs of the disorder are appearing in the unborn fetus and the newborn, but Vitamin B_6 deficiency *can*. And we know exactly what Vitamin B_6 deficiency does to blood vessels, because we've had it tested by the largest group of (unknowing) guinea pigs in history—the women who took the birth control pill. In carefully controlled studies involving 46,000 women, it has been demonstrated that the Pill causes deficiency in this vitamin and that deaths from vascular (blood-vessel) diseases are *40 times* greater in the Pill takers than in nonusers.

Thanks in part to our psychotic food-processing techniques, excessive losses in cooking, increased need for vitamin B_6 as we age, and greatly increased requirements for those on oral contraceptives, we have a national lack of the vitamin. And that's only a fragmented view of the influence of pregnancy nutrition on the next generation. But to return to the subject of nutrition as a weapon against difficulties in reproduction, a conversation I had with a veterinarian-nutritionist is pertinent. (That's probably redundant—vet schools *always* give numerous courses in nutrition; medical schools *usually* don't. They don't even have time for sex education, for heaven's sake!) I described for the vet the regimen nationally prescribed by the obstetrical establishment for women deemed, accurately or not, to be candidates for pregnancy toxemia and eclampsia, two dreaded and sometimes deadly complications of pregnancy. I told the veterinarian, "They use a low-calorie, low-protein, low-salt diet, plus doses of a diuretic" (waterpill, in the vernacular of the menstruating woman). "Would you be willing to prescribe that regime for a cow with pregnancy problems?" I asked. "Hell, no," said the animal doctor. "A cow is worth a thousand bucks!"

My friend Dr. Tom Brewer has fought a lifetime battle with the establishment in obstetrics trying to outlaw this deadly practice, which, he flatly vows, causes the very troubles it is supposed to prevent. So far, he's won his battle vis à vis diuretics: the FDA finally yielded and made the manufacturers warn the doctors that diuretics are not to be used in pregnancy. And a few more malpractice suits should dampen enthusiasm for the diet. One such suit, based on the birth of a severely retarded and nearly blind little girl produced by a mother plied with the fruit-rice-low-salt-diuretic regime for what proved to be a nonexistent pregnancy problem, has already been settled in favor of the mother and child.

As for the childless: when I was a guest on the Mike Douglas program, he asked me for a biographical note of interest with which to introduce me. I suggested that he tell the audience that I had just attended a luncheon meeting of 227 families, all formerly infertile, who had achieved parenthood after acting upon the dietary hints in my broadcasts and books. Mike didn't label me as a nutritional godfather but as the *father* of 227 children, which earned for me the palpitating admiration of his audience. Actually, I don't know how many such children have been born to formerly infertile families, but I did have a note from one of them, celebrating the fourth newcomer in five years. The father asked a pointed question: "How do you turn it off, Doc?" Which doesn't make good nutrition a panacea for infertility, but a sadly neglected possible help. Years ago, scientists at Loma Linda University in California investigated this thesis and wound up with the conclusion that the usual therapy, hormone medication, if given without nutritional correction, represents "dropping seeds into unfertilized soil." It remains unfertilized to this day. And among the small band of physicians who do respect the role of better nutrition for better reproduction, there is still a tendency to concentrate principally on the woman's pregnancy diet. It not only takes two to tango, but there is (neglected) evidence that the father's diet before conception may potently influence both his fertility and the fitness grade of the baby subsequently born. So it is that in an earlier book I offered a diet-supplement regime intended for both would-be parents, to be used long before conception is attempted. Indicating how the public's attitude is still shaped by current medical philosophy, that is the chapter which has drawn the fewest inquiries from readers. Which is passing strange, when you realize that a woman's chance of drawing a young mate who can't father children is one in six and, assuming a fertile husband, her chances of a disastrous pregnancy may be as great as one in four.

Inability to conceive isn't the only feminine problem for which nutrition may be an effective, if neglected, aid. Consider this note from one of my university students, who applied what she had learned in a classroom discussion of diet versus premenstrual tension and the painful menstrual:

"Dear Professor Fredericks," she wrote. "I am writing you to thank you for telling the class about Vitamin B Complex and menstrual periods. I was a student in your class last semester, and decided to try the B Complex because I suffered terribly each month. I used to have diarrhea, vomiting, and severe cramps every time. I had gone to a gynecologist who suggested three things: birth-control pills, dilatation [D & C], or have a baby. Due to the fact that none of these choices was very much to my liking, I continued to suffer. I even tried diuretics and pain killers, but nothing helped. That was until I started with the B Complex. I don't know how to thank you enough. I can't believe the difference. It feels really great not to have to go through that anymore. I only wish I had heard about it ten years ago. I also take multiple vitamins along with the B Complex. They have helped me tremendously. I'm really glad I took your course because it has not only helped me with the menses, but it has also helped me to have a better outlook and understanding about foods, nutrition, and health. Here's wishing you well. Sincerely, A.G."

The classroom discussion brought to my students the realization that premenstrual tension, backache, cramps, water retention, sensitivity of the breasts, irritability, fainting spells, and a prolonged menstrual with heavy hemorrhaging aren't normal but average, and may result from Vitamin B Complex deficiency. These vitamins are vital to the liver in controlling the activity of estrogen (female hormone). If the estrogen isn't kept at normal physiological levels, it may not only cause menstrual disturbances, but can be responsible for triggering cystic mastitis, uterine fibroid tumors, and estrogen-dependent cancer of the uterus and breast. Such breast cancers are one-third of the grim total. That means that insufficient intake of these B vitamins may pave the way toward troubles women usually accept as the *normal* price of being feminine. *Average*, yes; normal, no. Learn what my classes have been taught: when the premenstrual week drives women into asocial acts which invite jail sentences, or psychotic behavior which results in their being institutionalized, or attempts at suicide, there's nothing "normal" about the process.

One of my medical friends, reading the preceding paragraph, asked what specific signs of Vitamin B Complex deficiency I look for in fixing that as the cause of the estrogen misbehavior which leads to cystic mastitis, uterine fibroids, and estrogen-dependent cancer. My answer nonplussed him. "The cystic mastitis, the uterine fibroids, and the estrogen-dependent cancer *are* the symptoms of Vitamin B Complex deficiency." He protested. "That's sort of circular," he said. "And women are trapped in the circle," I shot back. Later he called me to say, "I found it difficult to believe that God put into the body of a woman a hormone which gives her everything from menstrual agony to breast cancer. And then I realized you weren't saying that. You were saying that the hormone causes trouble if the woman doesn't eat properly—and the Lord doesn't pick her menus."

The role of nutrition in breast and uterine cancer of the estrogen-dependent type has long been ignored by the cancer authorities, though they are aware that Japanese women, normally highly resistant to breast cancer, lose their immunity in about ten years after moving from Japan to Hawaii. Orthodoxy encounters a double problem in the thesis that nutrition provides the safeguard against the mischief of estrogen, for it involves not only the subject which medicine so long neglected—diet—but it also brings up the cancer-causing potential of a hormone which they've prescribed at the rate of $50 million worth yearly. To accept the proposition that Vitamin B Complex deficiency may turn estrogen—whether of external origin or produced by the ovaries—into a killer is to accept double culpability, for the profession not only shut its eyes to the carcinogenicity of estrogen, but has discouraged the public's use of vitamin supplements.

Perhaps my feelings would not be so obviously strong if I were not aware of the intellectual and scientific bankruptcy of the cancer establishment. How else would you characterize a medical specialty which views without reproach the "prevention" of breast cancer by the removal of noncancerous breasts? The excuse for a bilateral mastectomy in a noncancerous woman is the presence of a "risk" factor, which might be anything from breast cysts to a history of breast cancer in the family. One must say that it's effective—it's very difficult to develop breast cancer when you have no breasts. I know of ninety-two such operations, one of them on a fourteen-year-old, and that is the count for just three surgeons; there must be thousands more. The philosophy also includes hysterectomies, with oophorectomies (complete removal of uterus and ovaries). Like the Vitamin B Complex, this also reduces the body's estrogen load. One authority, committed to reducing the toll of breast cancer, has suggested that all women have such surgery at the age of thirty-eight. The comparable procedure, to reduce the incidence of prostate cancer, would be mass castration of all males at age, say, forty-five. Were the surgeons female, and making this proposal, do you think the men would be enthusiastic? If you think I am concerned with this exhibition of male chauvinism in a male-dominated medical specialty, you're right! But I'm more concerned about the women who do not realize that they must not so surrender their sovereignty over their own bodies.

In my own hometown, an oncological (cancer) surgeon performed a bilateral mastectomy on a fourteen-year-old girl, the excuse being that she came from a family prone to breast cancer. When criticized for such surgery on such a young child when she was perfectly normal, he darkly accused his opponents of favoring the death of the child from breast cancer. Aside from his monopoly on a crystal ball, one wonders whether the surgeon, who must be aware of the medical law of first do no harm, has reflected on what he has done to that little girl's future babies, who will necessarily be formula-fed and thereby lose the immunological protection afforded only by human breast milk. It is certainly the immunological system which, properly functioning, prevents us from universally being cancer victims.

To tame estrogen—whether in the birth control pill, prescribed for the menopause, or produced in excess by one's own ovaries—one encourages liver function by heightened intake of Vitamin B Complex, the nutritional antioxidants, and protein, accompanied by reduced intake of sugar. If a Vitamin B Complex supplement is used, it should provide generous amounts of choline and inositol. To get the biological antioxidants, it is necessary only to obtain a medical low-cholesterol diet and violate all its prohibitions, for these antioxidant factors are concentrated in eggs, liver, and other good foods banned in such a diet.

It is fortunate that the public is now aware of the cancer-producing potential of estrogenic hormone—medicine having ignored it for forty-five years. (Believe it: estrogen was known to cause eleven types of cancer in five species of mammals nearly a half-century ago, yet has been prescribed freely ever since.) The physician's defense is the contribution of estrogen to "improving the quality of life" for the menopausal woman. He is obviously the victim of effective estrogen advertising, which has persuaded him that the patient is locked into menopausal suffering sans estrogen therapy, or the risks of cancer with it. The following quotation from the JAMA (167:1806, 1958) should have dispelled that superstition: For a menopausal patient suffering from hot flushes in surgical menopause, Vitamin E was recommended in place of estrogen because it "had definite value in diminishing or causing absence of hot flushes."

I had promised myself that this book would not explore complicated areas of medicine and nutrition, but I must pause to tell you that, astonishingly, estrogen therapy for the menopause has been the subject of only one properly controlled, double-blind study, and *that* revealed that the placebo was as effective as the dangerous hormone. And if lack of estrogen is responsible for hot flushes, why don't little girls and all men, who are necessarily low in estrogen, have them? And why has removal of the uterus without removal of the ovaries still occasionally been followed by hot flushes? Suffice it to say that the medical nutritionist has much to offer the menopausal woman, and what he does carries no risks with it.

On the subject of adverse reactions to estrogen, up to and

95

including cancer, this note from a registered nurse is a striking example:

"Dear Doctor Fredericks: Thank God we women have someone like you to defend us. When you read an article such as the enclosed [recommending estrogen therapy for the menopause] you wonder what chance we women have with men such as this teaching in our medical schools.

"I survived in spite of a man like this—a highly respected OB-GYN [obstetrician-gynecologist] in Washington, D.C., also a teacher at a medical school there.

"Having been on estrogen two years, I began to have very slight, infrequent spotting. The Pap smears were negative. Being an R.N., I questioned him about the necessity of a D & C [dilatation and curettage]. He said not unless it became worse. In his opinion the spotting was insignificant, and caused by the estrogen.

"Thank heavens, a new M.D., after taking my history, said it *could* be caused by the estrogen, but the *only* way to really know was by having a D & C. To his astonishment and mine, a pathology report two pages long resulted. A hysterectomy was done, and everything turned out premalignant.

"My story had a happy ending. However, my present physician informed me that had I waited six months long, who knows? Had I not had the insight afforded me through being an R.N., I might not be alive to tell my story.

"This is *one* of the reasons your program is so valuable. Not only do you possess the knowledge to speak out, but, more importantly, the courage to speak out. Sincerely, Mrs. J.H.B."

Men also have troubles which are peculiar to their sex; the prostate is to the male what the breast is to the female. (There are some 60,000 cases of prostate cancer yearly, against 90,000 diagnosed cases of breast cancer.) Years ago, physicians experimenting with the administration of amino (protein) acids for a purpose unrelated to prostatitis were startled when some of the older patients in the group reported that their prostate troubles— urgency, burning, discomfort—had been sharply improved. The amino acids responsible for the improvement were identified and marketed—and the product was promptly taken off the market by the FDA. You will note that estrogen is still on the market.

Another problem, obviously unique to men, is a disease affecting the penis, described as one of the most painful disorders known. It's called Peyronie's disease. Consulted by a physician on possible nutritional therapies for the condition—for the medical resources are scant—I suggested that he try large doses of Vitamin E. The patient's response was slow but very gratifying, and in the course of his improvement, another disorder with which he suffered likewise responded. That is called Dupuytren's contracture, a strange illness in which the hand is drawn into a clawlike position. Surgery achieves a cosmetic improvement, but the hand then is virtually useless. About a year after that episode, I received a distressed letter from an old friend, a physician who had retired after many years of fine medical service, and was driven frantic when Dupuytren's contracture developed and interfered with the golf he had expected to enjoy in his well-earned years of rest. I told him about the single response I had seen, and urged him to try mixed tocopherols, a form of Vitamin E. Several months later he sent me a picture which needed no accompanying letter. He was playing golf again.

Shortly after that, I read an American Medical Association bulletin announcing that Vitamin E does nothing for man—it is, in fact, a vitamin in search of a disease. All of this perpetuation of the cultural lag must amuse Deke Slayton, the astronaut who was grounded because of heart irregularities, which didn't yield to medication, but disappeared when he began to take Vitamin B Complex and Vitamin E. Moreover, he took the vitamins only because he was subject to colds, not anticipating any therapeutic effect on his heart problem. It was obviously solved—he was in orbit not long after.

Which reminds me of a call I once got from an old friend, Dr. Sol Hirsch, who informed me that he had been hospitalized after a severe coronary thrombosis. What to do nutritionally, was the question. I had been a consultant for the doctor for many years, and pointed out that he knew what to do, but that didn't satisfy my old friend. I reeled off the list of nutrients important to the function of the heart, useful in stimulating collateral circulation, and helpful in reducing the need of the body for oxygen. The good doctor called his office and had the requisite supplements sent to his room. A week later his cardiologist walked in with the latest electrocardiogram and said, "Sol, no seventy-four-year-old man shows this kind of improvement after a severe coronary, and in any case, not in this short period of time. You must be doing something I don't know about." My naive medical friend admitted it, threw open the night table drawer, and showed the practitioner the array of supplements. His doctor's reaction was, at least, enigmatic. "If you're taking vitamins," he said, "I'm off your case." And he was. It was probably the most therapeutic move he had made for his patient.

And that episode was prelude to another, cut of the same fabric. A physician asked me for nutritional data concerning the treatment of angina, explaining that he had been forced to retire from practice because his heart condition was so debilitating that he had to use three nitroglycerin pills in sequence to allow him to ascend a flight of stairs. It was some months later that he wrote to say, "Last night, my wife stopped me as I was running upstairs to remind me that I have a heart condition." Subsequently, that physician wrote a chapter on heart disease for Dr. Morris Fishbein's *Home Medical Advisor.* I read it with pointed interest. Nowhere in it was there any mention of the possibility that harmless vitamin therapy might benefit sufferers from angina. This capitulation to the official party line was, I thought, to be expected—and to be regretted. The party line, incidentally, rejects nutritional therapy for heart disease such as angina on the basis of negative findings in "large-scale research" on 100 patients. It is offered to disprove Wilfred Shute's positive findings on a substantial percentage of more than 30,000 patients.

The contradictions in the cardiologists' dim view of nutrition in heart disease becomes apparent when one considers a disorder rather common in the elderly: intermittent claudication (lameness), which creates immobilizing pain when normal demands are made, such as in walking, on the muscles of the legs. The condition allows an objective measurement of benefits from any treatment, for one can measure walking distance without pain, before and after treatment. It is acknowledged in many medical papers that Vitamin E is an effective therapy for many cases of intermittent claudication, which means that the vitamin treatment has obviously rectified a metabolic disturbance of the leg muscles. The heart, I need not remind you, is a muscle, too, and, in heart disease, certainly a target for metabolic disturbances. In fact, what I have just written is a description of the coincidence which convinced my old friend Dr. Wilfred Shute that Vitamin E has a potential for the treatment of angina. He had given the vitamin to a patient, a barber, who had intermittent claudication and also suffered from angina. His legs responded. So did his heart, and the Shute brothers went on to treat their more than 30,000 cardiac patients with Vitamin E. Their favorable findings were "refuted" by the American cardiologist who thoroughly tested Vitamin E therapy on 100 patients, not one of whom showed any benefit. May I tell you that 100 heart patients given a placebo—an inert capsule which they think is medication— will, in thirty cases in 100, show a favorable response to the power of suggestion? What was wrong in the experimental conditions when there was zero response in all the 100 subjects?

That isn't the only contradiction one can find in the cardiologists' stolid resistance to nutritional therapies in heart conditions. Consider the recent announcement from the University of Texas, where researchers report benefit in cardiac disease from administration of coenzyme Q. Omitted from the wire service story, as it was from the Texas release: Vitamin E, years ago, was found essential to the body's synthesis of the enzyme.

Which brings up the answer I sent to a cardiovascular specialist, head of that clinic at a major hospital, who had asked me for a diet that would improve tolerance for aspirin. His patient, twenty-eight years old, had had a bilateral amputation of both legs below the knee, for "premature atherosclerosis." The aspirin was needed to help prevent postoperative blood clots. My answer was brief. Quoting Dr. Alton Ochsner, who used Vitamin E to reduce the incidence of postoperative clotting and phlebitis (thrombophlebitis), a frequent complication after surgery, I remarked: "The natural anticlotting factor in human blood isn't aspirin. It's alpha-tocopherol-phosphate (Vitamin E)."

Some of the caution medical men exhibit when a nutritionist offers a new (to them) perspective on nutritional therapies in human disease is predicated upon an ancient axiom, taught in every medical school: Be not the first to lay the old aside, nor yet the last to adopt the new. But if you translate that literally, no physician would ever be guilty of innovation. That is the problem I faced some twenty years ago, of which I was reminded by a very recent note in my diary. I had given a lecture in Chicago, after which I was approached by a young woman who said: "I am your daughter." Somewhat shaken by the announcement, I pointed out that I had not been in Chicago twenty years ago. She explained:

"My mother was seriously ill with ulcerative colitis in Medical Center in New York, and she was getting worse, though they'd tried every treatment short of surgery. She persuaded her doctor, who was head of gastroenterology, to call you for a suggestion. You suggested large doses of dried colon tissue, which sounded to him like the witch doctor philosophy—eat brains to be wise, eat heart to be courageous, and eat colon for a sick colon. Because he felt that mother might not survive, he tried the treatment, and it worked. But when she was discharged, he warned her never to become pregnant because, he said, that might reawaken the ulcerative colitis. She decided to go on taking the powdered colon tissue *and* to have a baby. That's me. So I'm your daughter."

The fascinating aspect of that history is the origin of my recommendation, which I didn't pluck out of the blue. Vacuum-dried colon tissue had been recommended for ulcerative colitis in proprietary advertising in a number of medical journals for many years.

Some of my consultations with dentists have provided grateful relief from the cynicism with which the nutritionist has been greeted over the years by other professions. A typical note in my diary concerns the little boy with the vast appetite for Danish pastry. His dentist called me with a genuine puzzle. The youngster's gums were a classic exhibit of Vitamin C deficiency in an advanced stage: there was spontaneous bleeding from the mere pressure of the pillow on his cheek as he slept. The practitioner had prescribed 100 m.g. Vitamin C daily, which in pre-Linus Pauling days was considered a fair dose. There had been no response, and yet the dentist insisted the diagnosis was correct. At his request I interviewed the patient, and stumbled on an interesting admission. He worked as an errand boy for a bakery shop where, at the end of the day, he was permitted to take home a bagful of sweet buns. Boys being boys, he arrived home with the sweet buns in the boy rather than in the bag—over a dozen of them. I called the dentist, cited the interplay between carbohydrate and Vitamin C, and offered two choices: reduce the sugar intake or increase the Vitamin C dose. The bleeding disappeared when the dose was raised. Sans the supplement, the boy's gums remained healthy when he lost his job.

The great Pasteur inflicted upon us a concept which for a century blinded us to the role of nutrition in the body's immune system. The Pasteur doctrine had it that we encounter a wandering bug and become infected. This ignores the fact that at this moment you probably have more than one such intruder in your body and yet are not infected, for the insult must fall upon a hospitable soil. That was the philosophy with which I approached another dentist's problem patient. The man, an Italian, had a case of Vincent's ulceromembranous stomato-gingivitis, a terrifying term for a terrifying attack of trench mouth. He had been treated with germicidal dyes, antibiotics, and ultraviolet irradiation, but the trench mouth, so painful that he had difficulty in swallowing saliva, persisted. The bacteria which are responsible for this type of infection are oxygen haters, which led me to the conclusion that his gums were oxygen poor, to put it unscientifically, and I recommended that the dentist treat him with the diet and vitamins which would ordinarily be used for a case of pellagra, including high protein, Vitamin B Complex, and heavy doses of niacinamide. The trench mouth yielded, but the patient was resistant to continuing on menus which omitted his usual gargantuan intake of pasta. He returned to his old dietary habits. He also returned to his old trench mouth, and the lesson was finally taught. The clue to all this was obvious, if overlooked: despite the classic infectiousness of this condition, he was the only member of his family with it. He was also the only member of the family who was stuffed with overprocessed carbohydrate.

Apropos of white flour and such, I once received recognition which to me is a more signal than a Nobel Prize: I was the subject of a cartoon in the funny papers! In it, a little boy comes home from school and tells his mother, "I swapped my Carlton Fredericks whole-wheat, wheat-germ, high-protein, vitamin-stuffed sandwich for Eddie's peanut-butter-and-jelly-on-white bread." His mother remarks that Eddie must have thought the nutritious sandwich pretty good, if he was willing to swap. "Nope," says the little boy, "I had to throw in my stamp collection and my ten-speed bicycle."

II
A Nutritionist's
Materia Medica

7

Using Nutrition Against Illness

In backlash against the dogmas of medicine, and against the failures and side reactions of conventional medication, my listeners and readers turn to nutrition, demanding immediate cures or at least immediate relief from their sicknesses. In the very nature of nutrition versus disease, both these are unlikely.

They also want me, a Ph.D., to diagnose and prescribe, by telephone at my office, via two-way radio, by mail, or in direct response to desperate questions from lecture audiences. However, although orthodox medicine has ignored nutrition in its training and rejected it in its practices, the laws define therapeutic nutrition as a facet of the practice of medicine, which is thereby legally denied to a Ph.D. Yet were I an M.D., what you are seeking would be difficult, impossible, or at best, unethical: who can competently treat a person without accurate diagnosis, without medical and nutritional history? The usual response when I point this out is an indignant, "But this is an emergency! And nutrition isn't medicine!" Unfortunately for this thesis, there are vanishingly few emergencies in nutrition, for a triumph of such therapy is usually a monument to needed but neglected changes in your dietary habits of long age. *Anything* used for the treatment of a disorder—even water—legally becomes a medicine, and recommending it is the practice of medicine. I *know*. This legal fiction, applied to a recommendation of a multiple vitamin supplement, was used in an effort to silence my broadcasts years ago.

In writing this part of the book, therefore, I am torn among motivations that are often squarely opposed. The overriding consideration I have already shared with you: in years as a clinical nutritionist, working with physicians and as a consultant to the professions, I have learned how to use food and food factors as adjunct or prime treatment in many disorders for which drug therapy is useless, ineffective, dangerous, or at best, productive of nothing more than relief of symptoms; and I don't want to take that information with me when I retire, or, unforgivably, die. And that's not a joke. My mail tells me that people have not yet forgiven Adelle Davis for her death, as if poor nutrition were the only cause of cancer and good nutrition an unfailing protection against it. It is as if nutritionists are not permitted illness, certainly not a fatal one.

I don't want to encourage self-medication, either, for anything more serious than the common cold. I know that you're impatient with that philosophy, all the more so because of your difficulties in finding physicians who are competent nutritionists. But self-treatment carries with it too many dangers. You may not be treating what you think you are. You may have something else wrong, of which you are unaware, and which will then be neglected. Example: the B Complex factor, PABA, occasionally restores pigmentation to the skin in the harmless disorder called "vitiligo". But vitiligo may be the unthreatening symptom under which hides lack of stomach hydrochloric acid or any one of a half-dozen other not-so-harmless disorders.

Another risk is failure to recognize the need or the opportunity profitably to raise or lower doses. Or you may bypass the need to employ other useful—or even vital—treatments, including the use of nutrients other than those I employ.

Conversely, a most powerful motive for writing what you are about to read lies in the possibility that your physicians are locked into orthodox drug therapies, and regard nutrition and nutritionists as suspect. Let me illustrate that point with the history of a twenty-one-year-old girl who was a graduate of a childhood of psychotic episodes and asocial behavior. She was now labeled hopelessly schizophrenic, and her despairing parents were being prodded into consenting to subject her to "psychosurgery," which is the medical title for an operation which makes patients manageable by making them something less than human beings.

In their anguish, the girl's parents sought alternative and less drastic treatments, but were relentlessly pressured by their psychiatrist, who pictured the brain operation as the unavoidable, last-ditch, and only possible solution to their endless problems with their daughter. The family doctor was not convinced of this, though, and suggested that the parents investigate psychonutrition. They resolved to send their daughter to the North Nassau Mental Health Center in New York where such orthomolecular psychiatry has rescued thousands of schizophrenics. The psychiatrist who had recommended brain surgery was outraged. In essence, he was saying: "Assault the brain surgically? Yes! Diet and vitamins? No!" Fortunately, the family ignored his advice, and their daughter is now well—one of 8,000 such patients who have profited from psychonutrition at that one center. Which makes it fascinating that the American Psychiatric Association, whose philosophy was guiding the surgery-minded psychiatrist and whose members had failed to help those 8,000 schizophrenics, has condemned the nutritional treatment of schizophrenia as valueless.

Another history, which I owe to Dr. William Philpott, is that of a pair of identical twins, both of whom were autistic. Diagnosis was established by a neurologist at Albert Einstein School of Medicine in New York. Neither twin could converse, neither could be educated, and both were markedly hyperactive. Dr. Philpott found the twins deficient in a number of nutrients, in virtually the same degree. He found them allergic to six foods, any one or any combination of which touched off their brain allergies, fanning the hyperactivity. Withdrawal of these foods from their diet caused the hyperactivity to disappear and, in addition, allowed the twins to communicate with each other and with their parents and teachers. In short, they became educable.

The neurologist who had diagnosed their condition called the mother, as he did at intervals, to ask her to bring the twins to a medical conference at Einstein. As identical twins with identical autism they were prime exhibits of the genetic factor in the disease. When she told him that the boys were no longer hyperactive, were communicating, were being educated, and that all this had been accomplished by correcting their deficiencies and withdrawing the foods to which they were allergic, the neurologist said, and I quote, "But that's not scientific. You have to do a double-blind study." He meant that it was possible that the twins had responded to the power of suggestion rather than to the nutrients and the hypoallergenic diet. Question: autistic children by the very nature of the disorder don't respond to suggestion or anything else. You can't reach them. How could they have responded to suggestion?

I cite the incident as a classical example of what happens when official doctrine replaces common sense in a highly trained physician. I cite the case histories and I write this section of the book to be sure that you make your decisions on the basis of a full understanding of an alternative kind of healing: nutrition. That understanding, though, doesn't dilute the advantages of obtaining competent medical guidance in applying the information in this book, though I know that some of you will protest: "My doctor is down on diets and vitamins!" Again, we tend to be down on what we're not up on, which is to say that the physician with that negative philosophy isn't competent in nutrition and refuses to admit it.

I have anticipated that problem by giving you at the end of the book the names of medical societies which concentrate on holistic medicine, and thereby on nutrition.* (Consulting medical nutritionists doesn't mean that you must discard your personal physician. You are entitled—always—to a consultation. The general practitioner who disqualifies himself in radiology by sending you to a radiologist, in gynecology by sending you to a gynecologist, or in psychiatry by sending you to a psychiatrist

*See Appendix B: A Listing of Competent Practitioners.

must abdicate his attitude of infallibility in nutrition too, if he's not entitled to wear that crown.) If you write to any of them, enclose a stamped, self-addressed envelope, and be sure to specify the type of practitioner you are seeking. It will do little good if you land in the office of a proctologist who practices nutritional therapies when your problem is your eyesight. Ask for a list of practitioners in your general area, and be specific about whether you are requesting a medical nutritionist (which is equivalent to an internist or a general practitioner), an orthomolecular psychiatrist, a dentist practicing preventive dentistry, or whatever. You may not find a practitioner in your home area, for while the number of nutrition-oriented practitioners grows daily, it's a big country and there are many barren areas.

The term *holistic medicine* should be defined—or rather illustrated. If you have a skin rash, diarrhea, and episodes of psychosis, your orthodox physician may prescribe a cortisone cream for the dermatitis, a clay product for the diarrhea, and a tranquilizer for the psychosis. Your holistic physician would give you Vitamin B Complex, niacinamide, and a high-protein diet, because this is the proper treatment for pellagra, which is one of the few diseases, if there are any others, which can simultaneously cause dermatitis, diarrhea, and delirium.

In the discussion of therapeutic nutrition which follows, you will find reference to two levels of intake. The first is the recommended level when the nutrient is used, as nutrients should be, to maintain good health. This is stated as a range because of individual differences in nutritional needs and tolerances. I have not given specific levels of therapeutic intake, which are also stated as a range, because, as you will come to understand by the discussions which follow, there are good reasons to seek medical-nutritional guidance when food and nutrients are used to cure rather than prevent.

The dividends from such nutritional fortification of the body can be rewarding, and authentic information is sometimes hard to come by. A telephone call I received recently from a friend is a good example. In her fifties, she had decided to have plastic surgery for bagging under the eyes, and asked me for a list of the nutrients important in minimizing the trauma and scar tissue

109

and accelerating the healing. I supplied it, suggesting that she discuss the matter with her surgeon. He gave her the damning, half-hearted assent I've heard as often as the term "spontaneous remission" applied to a nutrition-induced recovery: "It won't do any good, but it won't do any harm." But when she returned to his office after the operation, and he found her without the bruises and black eyes he had warned were inevitable, and observed that her healing was remarkably advanced and scar tissue minimized, he said: "I've given zinc in some acne cases when I'm doing dermabrasion, but I never thought of giving it to the other surgical patients." Then he emphatically requested that she record everything she had taken, and the doses.

When I heard the story, I was ironically amused, for some years ago a certain physician had shown conclusively how zinc supplements accelerate healing after surgery, while Wilbur Shute had demonstrated that Vitamin E, taken by mouth and applied locally, minimizes scar tissue. And the value of Vitamin C and bioflavonoids in minimizing hematomas (black and blue marks) was once convincingly shown by a football coach, using players at Tulane University as his test cases. And there you have a few examples of what I mean when I tell you that the information in this book had to be recorded and must not depart the scene with me.

I didn't arrive at my conclusions, incidentally, solely by reading papers by medical nutritionists. (For one thing, you learn a great deal from *veterinarian* nutritionists; the food needs of animals, since they are costly, are extensively studied by that profession.) My years as a clinical nutritionist with the Shaler Lawton Foundation and the Watch Hill Sanitarium helped, too. So did my intimate acquaintance with hundreds of medical nutritionists from coast to coast and in a number of foreign countries with whom I have long been on a first-name basis. As I write, I am thinking of Dr. Harold Harper, a medical nutritionist, who is a pioneer in chelation, which is a method, described later, in Appendix C, of allowing some patients to escape expensive and dangerous bypass surgery for circulatory and heart disorders. I saw Dr. Harper after he had suffered very severe burns, and he invited me to guess how old the injuries were. I thought he had been burned about two months before, but the actual timing was eighteen days! The acceleration of the healing and the minimizing of the scar tissue were dividends from prompt, continued use of a high-protein diet with supplements of zinc, Vitamin C, Vitamin E, and bioflavonoids, plus local applications of Vitamin E to the burned areas. To my knowledge, other than the use of thirty-five egg yolks daily for burn patients in an Israeli hospital, that kind of nutritional treatment isn't in use anywhere in this country. Nor is it used in preparation for plastic or any other kind of surgery. I've already pointed out that the "accepted" preparation for surgery is starvation, garnished with intravenous sugar.

As I write, I am also conscious of unmentioned subjects. I'm thinking of a pneumonia patient, ninety-one years old and in coma, who remained in the hospital for twelve days before he died with a sudden heart block. During those twelve days, he was given an antibiotic and glucose (sugar) by vein. When asked to institute "hyperalimentation"—superfeeding by vein—the resident physician announced that the hospital didn't "believe in vitamins." Once again the credo appeared to be starvation rather than nutrition. When asked if he would have recommended a twelve-day fast for the ninety-one-year-old if he had been conscious, the doctor remained silent. I regard that death as iatrogenic, which means homicide by approved treatment.

The discussion in the chapters which follow doesn't cover all the hundreds of diseases to which the flesh is heir. Although there is *no* disease, however caused, which will not ultimately involve nutrition, if only at the cellular level, nutrition isn't a panacea. I confine myself to reporting what I know to be helpful, with cognizance of individual differences: there will be those who will respond magnificently and those who will not respond at all. In the observations which follow, a few will be new, not only to you, the reader, but to medical and nonmedical nutritionists. I do not apologize for observations and conclusions which are my own, though I must note that each of us in the health professions stands on the shoulders of those who have gone before.

It is both possible and probable that a book like this, written

111

twenty-five years from now, will record many other diseases in which nutrition will have been found useful in prevention, treatment, or both, and I make the safe prophecy that its author will voice his frustrations, as I have mine, over the resistance of the establishment to new ideas and the tenacity of the public in clinging to outworn concepts. Some of those ideas are now reflected in questions with which every nutritionist is faced: "What is the diet for arthritis? For schizophrenia? For autism?" Implicit in these questions is a fallacious assumption: that every disease is a single disorder, of a single origin, and thereby amenable to a single nutritional approach. And behind that is another fallacy: that we can consider the effect of the disease on the person without considering the effect of the person on the disease. (As one example of such a variable, consider the fact that a given disease is likely to be more severe in very tall and in very short people. The ideal height seems to be 5′ 10″—not by coincidence, *my* height.) The point is that we are biochemically more dissimilar than alike, and no generalizations can be made about our nutritional needs, whether in health or in sickness.

The multiple faces of the enemy—disease—are well illustrated in arthritis. The term is generic, covering rheumatoid arthritis, osteoarthritis, and hypertrophic, palindromic, psoriatric, menopausal, traumatic, Marie Strumpel, and several allied varieties. Diabetes is similarly a generic term, under which appear the juvenile type, the mature onset, the mature onset masquerading as juvenile, the allergic type, the type resulting from chromium deficiency, that caused with errors in the body's immune mechanisms, a viral type, and one in which the liver may play a more important role than the pancreas. The nutritionist would be no more justified in postulating a single nutritional approach to any of these than the physician would be in mimeographing his prescriptions.

Whatever the diseases and the types, there are certain common denominators which make possible some of the generalizations you will encounter in the pages which follow. Diabetics, for example, do share problems in the utilization of food factors, not only sugar, as lay legend has it, but protein, fat, vitamins, minerals, and, in one type, water. Whatever the origin of multiple sclerosis, the disease is marked by loss of the myelin insulating sheaths which protect the nerves, and treatment aimed at halting or reversing that process must be helpful. Whatever the chemistry of a particular autistic child, removing allergens from the diet must help; in certain types, Vitamin B_6 therapy will rectify a disturbance in the biochemistry of the child, and Vitamin E will sometimes be helpful. The hyperactive child and the schizophrenic child or adult, whatever their chemistries, will improve when a hypoglycemia is present, which it frequently is, and is controlled.

Having given you a few of the common denominators, let me point out that there are situations where they can't freely be invoked. Take, for instance, the case of a hypoglycemic whose low blood sugar is aggravated by multiple food allergies. If these are not identified, the diet which helps others with low blood sugar may fail to help him; it may even worsen his condition, for it is possible to be allergic to good foods as well as to sugar and caffeine. The nutritionist has an advantage over the prescriber of drugs, however: our "side reactions" are never lethal, seldom serious, and usually nothing more than intolerance.

What you have just read reaffirms the importance of competent medical supervision in the application of therapeutic nutrition. It underscores the admonitions which you will find in the pages which follow, where I emphasize taking full advantage of the preventive applications of nutrition, while seeking the counsel of medical nutritionists in applying the science as a treatment.

8

The Subject Is Pain:
Arthritis

If arthritis is the theme, the theme song is "Take aspirin and learn to live with it!" The medical bankruptcy reflected in that statement has been the cross borne by millions of sufferers with osteoarthritis and rheumatoid arthritis, the two most common types of these degenerative diseases. The physician's sparse resources for treating these painful, disabling disorders are matched by the limited responses of many of his patients. Moreover, the list of serious side reactions to some of his medications is so long as to raise serious questions concerning the risk-versus-benefit ratio.

In its approach to the most common types of arthritis, the medical profession is hampered by negative philosophies. The first of these is inherent in our medical system, for although we may call it health care, what we get is actually *sickness* care. The second is the attitude of cooperating with the inevitable, which becomes inescapable when osteoarthritis is labeled as a "wear and tear" disease. Wear and tear being as unavoidable as taxes and death, this means that we must all surrender to it; moreover, it is neither preventable nor amenable to cure. (Which doesn't explain why some of us don't develop osteoarthritis. Did we manage to escape wear and tear? Or did something—our nutrition, perhaps—protect us?)

114

In rheumatoid arthritis, we are faced with a medical view of the body as failing to recognize its own tissues and attacking them as if they were alien intruders. But treatment of rheumatoids isn't aimed at restoring sanity to an immune system which has lost its normal cues; it is largely symptomatic. So it is that medicine does its best, which is tragically often not good enough, to contain rather than to avoid or cure these diseases, and to keep the patient more comfortable. Which doesn't stop millions of arthritis sufferers from enduring pain, stiffness, reduced joint mobility, and impaired social and vocational functioning.

Conventional medical treatment for arthritis varies, depending both on the type and on the philosophy of the physician, but generally involves aspirin or other painkillers, anti-inflammation drugs, doses of cortisone or other steroid hormones, injections of gold or penicillamine, and prescriptions for exercise, physiotherapy, or rest. Less conventional treatment for pain uses hypnosis, biofeedback, and transcendental meditation. Blood dialysis (filtering) is in experimental use. Though a number of the drugs cause dangerous side reactions (penicillamine treatment, for example, must be withdrawn for one-third to one-half of the patients because of untoward effects), nothing in that list is frowned on by the arthritis establishment. What the Arthritis Foundation vehemently and totally disapproves is any attempt to prevent or to treat arthritis with nutrition. As you will realize when you have finished reading this discussion, this attitude is arbitrary, capricious, and based on the largest blind spot in the eyes of establishment medicine. When I read the foundation's blasts at "nutrition quackery" in arthritis, I am reminded of an axiom which pleases me because I invented it: ignorance is a challenge to an educator, but opinionated ignorance is a disaster. You'll appreciate the accuracy of that observation if you spend a few days in a medical library, where you can uncover many reports from competent clinicians who have benefited their arthritic patients with controlled diet and effective doses of appropriate nutrients. Which means that what follows isn't based on my personal theories. It derives from experience on the medical firing line— what medical nutritionists have learned by watching the responses of arthritis victims to therapeutic nutrition. And those responses range from slight relief of pain and stiffness to discarding of canes, crutches, and walkers.

The story begins with the reactions of cattle when, for want of normal feed, they are compelled to graze on weeds of the nightshade family. As a result of the toxicity of these plants they develop such severe pain in their joints that they will be found kneeling rather than standing normally. This phenomenon was observed by Dr. Norman F. Childers, Blake Professor of Horticulture at Rutgers University, New Brunswick, New Jersey. The professor was suffering with a severe arthritis which had, as it so often does, appeared out of the blue, and he was searching for the explanation, which his physician could not offer. Dr. Childers was aware that his own diet, like that of so many Americans, contained many foods from the nightshade family, which includes all the peppers save black pepper, and tomato, white potato, and eggplant. (Professors of horticulture usually have access to experimental gardens where such crops are grown.) The professor wondered whether the toxic effects of the nightshades on the joints of cattle had any parallel in human beings. He avoided those foods. His arthritis vanished as it had appeared, and Dr. Childers was propelled into a decade of research on the role of the nightshade plants in causing arthritis in the susceptible. I must emphasize that last term: in the *susceptible*, for many of us eat nightshade plants without penalty, and many arthritics can't blame their troubles on that plant family. But millions *can*, as the professor demonstrated in more than ten years of study of thousands of arthritics. Not only were they benefited, some to the point of freedom from the disease, but a number of them who decided after they were cured to return to eating the nightshades had an astonishingly quick return of symptoms.

The Arthritis Foundation's reactions to this decade of research were predictable. "At best, the announcement is premature," said the high priests of inactivity. "At worst, it's false." As the writer and broadcaster who brought Dr. Childers' findings to the public, I responded with, "At best, the Arthritis Foundation's statement is premature, and at worst, it is false." I had, you see, already received a number of letters from radio listeners and readers who had abandoned the nightshade plants and achieved relief from arthritis.

The history goes beyond this: some of the nightshade-sensitive also suffer depression when they eat these plants. Some develop diverticulosis. And, in recent research at the U.S. Department of Agriculture, there is a hint that the nightshades may contribute to heart trouble. (One is almost compelled to be reminded that the introduction of the potato in the European diet met with determined resistance, for there was a "superstition" that this was not a food good for human beings. The term "spud" for potato is supposed to have originated with the Society for Prevention of Unnutritious Diet, SPUD).

Avoiding the nightshades is troublesome, for they are ingredients in many dishes. Paprika, for example, is ubiquitous as a seasoning. Peppers find their way into many pre-prepared dishes. Avoiding tomato will ban more than ketchup and virtually all favorite Italian recipes. Reading labels *very* carefully is the only way to stay on a diet free of nightshades. Do remember that not all arthritis is owed to sensitivity to these plants, and even when it is, it may take months before the benefits appear. Age, happily, is no barrier to response.

From his fellow horticulturists, Dr. Childers met with opposition even more blind and dogmatic than that of the Arthritis Foundation. His peers did not, as scientific custom and decency would dictate, listen to his papers and then let loose with a barrage of (untested) objections. They actually attempted to keep him from *reading* his papers anywhere. If this is at odds with your picture of the way scientific discoveries are normally greeted, remember that many university horticulturists are closely linked with the agribusiness complex, via grants, endowments, and consultation relationships. Their behavior, though inexcusable, can be explained if you remember the ancient saying "Whose bread I eat, his song I sing." Substitute nightshade plant for bread, and you update the saying. Despite the opposition, Dr. Childers has persisted in his research, now involving more than 5,000 arthritics who correspond with him, giving reports in great detail. (One of them is a horticulturist who was originally among Childers' bitterest critics.) Dr. Childers knows he's right, and so do I, and so do the patients who benefited from his findings.

In vitamin therapy for osteoarthritis, a significant discovery was made some thirty years ago. The physician responsible for it, Dr. William Kaufman, was like Dr. Childers a friend of mine. He didn't meet the opposition the horticulturist faced; he was simply ignored. I encountered his papers almost casually, and was so impressed by their importance to arthritics that I not only made it a point to meet with Dr. Kaufman, but was responsible for bringing his research to the attention of the International Academy of Preventive Medicine, which honored him with the Tom Spies Award.

Dr. Kaufman and Dr. Childers followed paths which were in a measure parallel. The horticulturist observed the joint pain in cattle grazing on nightshades. The medical man was aware of joint pain in patients with pellagra, and thereby decided in essence to apply the nutritional therapy for pellagra to arthritis. Ultimately, he learned that a good diet, supplemented with generous amounts of niacinamide far beyond the postulated "daily requirement," was very effective in the treatment of osteoarthritis, and could be applied in some of the rheumatoids too, for there is often a mixture of the two diseases. He found, too, that—just as in pellagra—some arthritis patients also benefit by dosage with other vitamins of the B Complex.

Although I usually avoid expanding on personal experience, what I encountered personally with application of Dr. Kaufman's research is worth describing. I was once involved in a serious accident in which I received neck and back injuries which were silent for a long time but eventually exploded as a traumatic arthritis. I avoided the dispensers of cortisone and aspirin and obtained osteopathic and chiropractic manipulation, which reduced but didn't completely relieve the stiffness and the flashes of intense pain. After reading Dr. Kaufman's monograph on niacinamide treatment of osteoarthritis, I was impressed with his objective appraisals of his clinical results. They had brought him such quiet fame among arthritis sufferers that a letter addressed to The Arthritis Doctor, Bridgeport, Connecticut, was promptly delivered to him. By "objective appraisals" of his patients' responses, I mean that Dr. Kaufman used two gauges of the improvement of his osteoarthritis patients. One of these was a "joint range index" which allowed him to determine objectively to what extent the patients recovered mobility of the joints. The other was a simple device to measure the strength of muscles, which are often weakened in osteoarthritics. By both standards, his niacinamide treatment had significantly benefited thousands of such patients. It did the same for me, which is doubly interesting because I was taking that vitamin, among others, long before I encountered Dr. Kaufman, but raising my intake from 50 mg. daily to 125 mg. brought a remarkable relief from stiffness and pain. In some three years at that level of dosage, which brings the history to the present date, I have had only two fleeting episodes of the pains which once were previously daily companions.

Ultimately, Dr. Kaufman was able to demonstrate that a good diet, supplemented with amounts of niacinamide considered huge in the forties and fifties, was effective for treating both osteoarthritis and cases of rheumatoid arthritis in which the two types are mixed. He also found that it sometimes is necessary and helpful to employ doses of other B Complex vitamins. Yet the scholarly papers in which this physician reported on his lifelong research have received the usual neglect by the arthritis establishment. I might note, for the benefit of the scientifically trained, that what the therapy does *not* do is raise the pain threshold, which would make it a palliative painkiller, replacing aspirin. It actually appears to hold the process of degeneration at bay, and in some cases clearly to reverse it.

When Dr. Kaufman mentioned the added benefits from doses of other B vitamins, I was aware that his observation was one which crossed the research path of another medical nutritionist, Dr. John Ellis, who had observed a remarkable improvement in an arthritic who had been snacking on large amounts of pecans. Experiments determined that the Vitamin B_6 and potassium supplied by the nuts were responsible for the effect, which led this physician to treat thousands of osteoarthritics (he uses another

119

term, hypertrophic arthritis) with high doses of the vitamin and moderate supplements of potassium. (Potassium supplements really must not be used without medical guidance; they can be dangerous.) Dr. Ellis has restored thousands of patients to vocational and social functioning. His work has been, as usual, ignored by the arthritis establishment.

Dr. Ellis's research, involving yet another Vitamin B Complex factor, neatly coincided with another investigation reported by British physicians. They had observed that blood levels of pantothenic acid, which is important to adrenal gland function, were low in rheumatoid arthritics. Dosing with the vitamin to raise blood levels brought significant benefit to some patients, but something seemed to limit those levels, no matter how high the dose of the vitamin. Trying to break through that barrier, they employed "royal jelly," the food reserved by bees for larvae destined to become queen bees. Royal jelly is the richest natural source of pantothenic acid, and thereby might also contain factors synergistic with (working with) the vitamin. So it proved: oral doses or injections of royal jelly, coupled with supplements of pantothenic acid, raised the blood level beyond the invisible barrier they had encountered, and benefits to rheumatoid arthritics increased. This is doubly fascinating, for an uneven tide of production of adrenal hormones has been indicted as a contributing factor in causing rheumatoid arthritis, and pantothenic acid deficiency is known to interfere with the function of the gland. It has been demonstrated conclusively that supplementing pantothenic acid raises the body's resistance to stress, which is one of the key functions of the adrenal glands.

Zinc supplementing was also recently found to be helpful to rheumatoid arthritics. The use of this metal joins that of all the vitamins in being condemned as useless and quackery, on the basis of no organized evaluation at all.

There are painful disorders, sometimes associated with arthritis, sometimes occurring independently, which have also responded to nutritional therapies. Myositis, or painful muscles, bursitis, which causes pain and dysfunction in joints, and fibrositis, another painful muscular condition, are examples. In

120

my personal research, Vitamin E in the form of mixed toco-pherols, accompanied by local applications of wheat-germ oil ointment, has proved helpful in some of these disorders. The report on this wheat-germ oil ointment therapy was published by a physician nearly thirty years ago; it too has been ignored. Like the findings with the nightshades, niacinamide, Vitamin B_6 and potassium, royal jelly and pantothenic acid, it has been condemned—without testing, of course—as "nutritional quack-ery." One gets the feeling that were a vitamin discovered to-morrow and demonstrated to wipe out *all* arthritis, the arthritis establishment would ignore or outlaw it. Incidentally, it is fas-cinating that a factor of the Vitamin B Complex has been ad-vertised for myositis and other "arthritic" pain-causing conditions for years—and in the medical journals at that. But it isn't de-scribed as a vitamin. It's called the potassium salt of para-amino-benzoic acid, or PABA—which is found in every concentrate of Vitamin B Complex from natural sources. It *does* help some painful disorders of muscle and joint. And it *is* prescribed. Wait until they realize it's a vitamin! (At the time these lines are written, the FDA is considering a regulation which, among other prohibitions, will remove PABA from the market entirely.)

You may have read Norman Cousins's *Anatomy of an Illness* (New York: W. W. Norton, 1979), the story of his battle with ankylosing spondylitis, an "incurable" type of deforming arthritis. If you did, you learned that megavitamin doses of Vitamin C, plus generous amounts of laughter, constituted his self-prescrip-tion for his condition. He conquered it, and has since addressed numerous medical societies, written on the subject for at least one major medical journal, and is now lecturing about it at the U.C.L.A. medical school. One wonders if his audiences are (a) moved to consider large doses of Vitamin C in treating this condition, and (b) inspired to consider that Vitamin C stimulates the immune system, which in rheumatoid arthritis is certainly not functioning properly.

Dr. Joseph Broadman was a specialist in bee-venom therapy for arthritis, a treatment inspired by repeated reports that bee-keepers, who are stung frequently, have a striking immunity to these diseases. The Arthritis Foundation (as usual, without testing) called him a quack. They had picked on the wrong man, for fortified by the certainty that he had helped thousands of patients with bee-venom treatment, he sued for libel. The case was discreetly settled out of court, but no further papers appeared on the subject for many years, and it may be that the resistance of the establishment has once again interred another useful treatment. Here again I write from personal knowledge, for one of the medical nutritionists with whom I trained as a youngster kept a beehive in his office and used the stings of live bees to treat some of his arthritic patients.

Years ago, there was a study in which extra eggs were found more effective than the usual penicillin treatment in severe cases of rheumatic fever. I've seen excellent responses in adults with rheumatoid arthritis who were fed extra eggs as a part of a high-protein diet that was low in sugar and other processed carbohydrates, and properly supplemented with niacinamide, Vitamin E, zinc, and Vitamin C. It may be that the histidine (an amino acid, one of the building blocks of protein) which is richly supplied by eggs may be the key factor, for this amino acid has been used helpfully in the treatment of this type of arthritis. But we'll lack certain knowledge until the arthritis establishment relinquishes its stranglehold on orthodox medical thinking.

These therapies have common characteristics: they were developed by physicians at least as competent as their critics, and both the researchers and their research have been ostracized by the medical men wedded to cortisone, gold, and aspirin "therapy." This I tell you with all the conviction at my command: if I were in trouble with rheumatoid or osteoarthritis, I'd consult a medical nutritionist. And if I were a medical specialist in the arthritic disorders, every patient would be tested for sensitivity to (or intolerance of) the nightshade foods. (There is a simple test, based on weakening of indicator muscles when the person is exposed to the food.) And no patient would leave my office without providing a nutritional history, without undergoing tests for nutritional chemistries and for allergy, and without prescriptions for niacinamide, the Vitamin B Complex, mixed tocopherols (E), Vitamin C, zinc, pantothenic acid, royal jelly, and, if needed, wheat-germ oil ointment.

I cannot help thinking, as I write these lines, of a young man of twenty-eight who was in a wheelchair with rheumatoid arthritis and left the wheelchair after such nutritional treatment. He is now sixty-one and has never had a relapse. The explanation by his mystified doctor, who followed the dietary suggestions blindly, was "spontaneous remission." What else? I also think of one of my university students who is now a volunteer worker at the Fryer Foundation. Two years ago, she was literally crippled with rheumatoid arthritis. Indeed, when she announced that she was seeking a medical nutritionist, her physician pleaded with her husband to "straighten her out." Without cortisone and aspirin, he warned, he could not be responsible for what would happen to her, but hopeless crippling was inevitable. I have urged her, since her recovery on nutritional therapies, to revisit her physician, for he was obviously honestly concerned and honestly believed his warnings of doom. I had a surreptitious motive, of course: there was just a small chance that he might not consider her improvement to be a "spontaneous remission," and thereby might learn from the experience.

A nutritional prescription for arthritis patients should include the following ranges of supplementary intake:

Zinc. Should be used in the chelated form. From 10 mg. to 30 mg. daily.

Vitamin B$_6$ (pyridoxin). From 5 mg. to 50 mg. daily.

Vitamin E. Should be used in the form of mixed tocopherols. From 100 mg. to 200 mg. daily, measured in terms of alpha tocopherol potency. The elderly may need up to 400 mg. daily.

Niacinamide. Should not be used in the form of niacin, which causes flushing and does not have the protective effect of the "amide" form. From 50 mg. to 100 mg. daily.

Vitamin C. From 250 mg. to 2,500 mg. daily. Those on a low-salt diet should not use the sodium ascorbate form. Those sensitive to nightshades must check their reactions to concentrated Vitamin C. Some are intolerant of it in supplemental form.

PABA. 50 mg. daily.

Pantothenic acid. 50 mg. to 100 mg.

Potassium. Safely supplied by such foods as bananas, nuts, figs, raisins, and, if not sensitive to nightshades, tomato juice.

Royal jelly. Capsules containing fresh, rather than desiccated (dried), should be available. Supplementary dose is suggested by the manufacturer, since the quantity in the capsule varies from one maker to another.

9

Fewer Calories = Weight Loss?
Only in the Textbooks!

There is a law of thermodynamics which says that energy can neither be created nor destroyed. Translated in terms of body weight, it means that eating more than you need will make you store fat, and eating less will make you lean.

There's only one trouble with a law of physics when it is applied to energy metabolism in human beings. Laws don't vary, but human beings do, and energy pathways aren't the same in all people.

If eating fewer calories than you "burn" is the simple, effective solution to weight problems, why do we have Weight Watchers, TOPS, behavior modification specialists trying to change eating habits, diet pills, fat doctors, fat clinics, reducing spas, and a score of "new" reducing diets every year? Why do we have people who've lost a 1,000 pounds, 20 off, 20 on, year after year for a quarter of a century? Why do we have the obese who submit to having their jaws wired so that they must live on a liquid diet, and why are there overweight persons who surrender to surgeons, and let them remove part of their intestines in a deliberate attempt to create poor absorption of food?

And why do we ignore the patent fact that there are people whose weight gain is all out of proportion to their calorie sins, and those who overeat and escape weight penalties? Isn't the converse also true? Aren't there millions of (neglected) underweight people who should gain by eating more calories than they expend, but must nonetheless struggle to put on and retain a few needed pounds?

I should like to propose some answers to these questions. That becomes possible only if we recognize that the old ideas about the calorie equation don't work, because energy metabolism in the human body isn't a simple process, isn't uniform from person to person, and isn't a matter of burning calories versus storing them as fat. In this chapter, I will give you four different approaches to solving the weight problem. As it isn't feasible to set up a recommended dietary allowance (RDA) of nutrients to meet the differing requirements of millions of people whose biochemistries are anything but uniform, so is it unrealistic to assume that the single step of restricting total calorie intake will solve everyone's fat storage problems.

If eating too many calories makes you store the excess energy as fat, then the equation should (and is supposed to) work in reverse: eating too few calories should make you draw on your fat deposits for the missing energy. For some people, the theory works. For many, it's the wrong approach. Moreover, if it did work for everybody, then total starvation or fasting, the greatest calorie-deficient diet of all, should efficiently burn body fat. It doesn't. We know that with insufficient calories or with total fasting more than 60 percent of the weight loss occurs in tissues rather than body fat. It's protein we're burning, meaning that we're tearing down our own house. One needn't be an expert to realize that shrinking muscles, livers, and kidneys is not a step toward the better health promised to those who try to normalize their body weight. On the contrary, it's a disaster—and the calorie theory doesn't predict it.

Even if fasting or very low calorie diets did what the theory predicts, they still wouldn't be a desirable way to lose weight. No method is effective if it doesn't retrain eating habits; and starvation, whether total or partial, doesn't reeducate. That is another of the fallacies in blitz diets, wiring of jaws, and surgery to produce malabsorption.

If fasting burns protein rather than fat deposits, what happens when you go to the other extreme and eat a high-fat, high-protein, low-carbohydrate diet? Experiments in this regard were conducted on a group of U.S. Navy Hospital volunteers. When they fasted, they lost 20 pounds in two weeks, but 13 pounds of the weight loss was from tissue or protein, and only 7 pounds from fatty deposits. The same group was then placed on a high-fat, high-protein, low-carbohydrate diet for two weeks. They lost less than while fasting—only 13 pounds—but more than 12½ pounds of that was fat!

Let's sum up what we've learned. A drastic reduction in calories, which is what severe diets and fasting represent, doesn't do what the theory predicts it should. Second, fat loss is certainly determined by the types of food eaten and not by the calorie intake. Third, which I can personally verify, it is possible to lose weight on a high-protein, high-fat, low-carbohydrate diet while eating amounts of food which, by the calorie theory, should promote gain rather than loss. Not only that, but repeated experiments have shown fat weight loss on low-carbohydrate diets when used by people who had never been able to reduce on the classical low-calorie diets. And fourth, even if you test two different kinds of the same foods in the same amounts—for instance, starch versus sugar—you find another assumption to be fallacious, for animals gain more weight on sugar than they do on identical amounts of starch. This is simply another view of the error behind the "food-exchange lists" for diabetics, which assume that you can substitute calorie-equal portions of any carbohydrate for any other. The fact of the matter is that the blood sugar response to rice isn't the same as it is to banana, nor can sugar be equated with bread, or cornflakes with potato, even though calorie values are identical.

This explains what many dieters have sworn to be true over the vehement objections of orthodox nutritionists: you can gain more weight on sugar than on starch, quantity for quantity. Dismissed as folklore, this belief has recently been confirmed by a new understanding of the functions of the fat cells in the body. Formerly thought of as more or less inert warehouses for fat deposits, these cells are now known to be biochemically very active. Among their capabilities is that of converting blood sugar into fat. To do this, they need help from two metabolites: a breakdown product of sugar (alpha glycerophosphate) and insulin. Supplies of the breakdown product and insulin will be higher in sugar eaters; conversion of sugar into fat will be more efficient. A low-carboydrate diet, severely restricted in sugar, will obviously help to avoid or minimize that conversion. The gradual conversion of protein into sugar will keep blood sugar levels high enough to meet the body's needs without the violent upsurge of the level which follows the eating of sugar and which encourages conversion of it into fat. The chemistry involved here is identical with that observed in people with low blood sugar, most of whom thrive when sugar intake is eliminated while protein and fat are raised.

A carefully controlled research project at the University of Wisconsin Medical School showed that the addition of a small amount of vegetable oil to a low-carbohydrate diet will step up the burning of stored body fat. The chemistry has been explored: the vegetable oil "tugs" at the stored fat and induces it to return to the metabolic furnace to be oxidized. This, rather than sugar, is the process which supplies energy to such organs as the heart, muscles, and kidneys.

The action of vegetable oil—polyunsaturated fat—in nudging stored body fat back into the body furnace explains why the low-carbohydrate, high-protein, high-fat diet supplemented with vegetable oil sometimes reduces inches all out of proportion to the loss in pounds. It often solves the problem of the "tires" at the midriff and the heavy upper arm or upper thigh, which usually don't yield to weight loss by the conventional method. This failure is understandable when you remember that these are fat deposits, and that conventional diets target protein tissues instead.

When faced with a high-fat, high-protein, low-carbohydrate diet, many reducers suddenly discover that they've been brainwashed by the low-cholesterol, low-animal-fat propaganda. I deliberately use the term *propaganda,* for this is not science, but an oversimplistic attempt to explain very, very complicated problems in heart and blood-vessel diseases. You may ask: will not a high-fat diet lead to hardening of the arteries and heart attacks? From hundreds of negative replies, let me cite a few:

1. A man and his wife share the same meals. If diet is *the* explanation for heart attacks, why is she immune up to the menopause?
2. Why are numerous primitive groups on high-fat, high-protein diets, like the Masai and the Mongolians, largely immune to heart disease?
3. Why was the celebrated cardiologist Dr. Paul Dudley White told in 1912, when he proposed to become a heart specialist, that no physician could live on such a lean practice? Weren't people eating butter, cream, eggs, and plenty of animal fat in 1912?
4. Why are there millions of people with high blood cholesterol who are resistant to heart disease and atherosclerosis? And more millions with normal blood cholesterol who manage to develop heart attacks?
5. Finally, why are there some twelve or fifteen well-controlled studies which have not been able to show a significant relationship between cholesterol blood levels and arterial or heart disease? One of these was reported by Michael De Bakey, who was able to find no meaningful relationship between blood cholesterol levels and the condition of the artery walls— which, it should be pointed out, he was able to *see*.

That list could be extended to several pages, but suffice it to say that the person who has abnormally high blood cholesterol or who is on a medically prescribed diet should, if overweight, obviously reduce—but under his physician's supervision. And let me finish by pointing out a glaring inconsistency. Until the evidence which has been reviewed in these pages, was collected, every conventional low-calorie diet was supposed to reduce you by burning your own fat to supply the missing calories for energy. And, whether you like it or not, *your* body fat is *animal fat.* So *every* reducing diet, in the standard theory, is a high-animal-fat diet.

Another useful characteristic of the low-carbohydrate weight-loss diet is its effect in reducing salt retention. Loss of weight can come to a standstill if you retain salt, for from the burning of fat water accumulates, and if you retain it because of salt retention, you don't lose. The medical approach to this problem isn't good medicine, for it treats the symptom, water retention, rather than the cause, salt retention. A low-carbohydrate diet thereby makes more sense than the use of a "water pill" (diuretic) because it discourages retention of both salt and fluid. It is so effective that it has been used in other disorders where edema (swelling of the tissues from fluid retention) is a problem.

Whether you're a candidate for the low-carbohydrate diet or you're one of those who can effectively reduce by modest cutting of calories, you'll still find appetite and weight control easier if you divide your three daily meals into more frequent smaller ones, each with a modest amount of efficient (animal) protein, which means meat, fish, fowl, cheese, eggs, yogurt, etc. (Which doesn't mean yogurt flawed by the adding of fruit preserves, so that it has more sugar calories than yogurt calories.)

How do you know if the low-carbohydrate diet is more likely to meet your needs? The first clue comes from your diet history: if you've been successful in losing weight on a standard 1,200-calorie diet, your biochemistry is conventional. If, however, you don't tolerate carbohydrates well, your decision is made for you. Carbohydrate intolerance may be indicated by susceptibility to tooth decay, large tonsils and adenoids, water retention in the premenstrual week, an addictive craving for sweets, hypoglycemia (low blood sugar), diabetes or prediabetes, quick weight gain with modest carbohydrate sprees, and the opposite—quick loss of weight with modest reduction of intake of starches and sugars.

My standard 1,200-calorie diet isn't an extreme one. Weight loss should be from one to two pounds per week—fast enough to keep you reasonably happy, slow enough to keep me from worrying. (I've lost some good friends who tried the "blitz" method.) My low-carbohydrate diet isn't a rigorous one either; it reduces sugar-starch intake about 60 percent below the level of that of the 1,200-caloric conventional reducing diet. There are, of course, diets which recommend more extreme carbohydrate reduction, but some people don't tolerate that well, and I prefer a more conservative approach. You will note that vitamin-mineral supplements are used with all my diets. The purpose is obvious: to protect you against deficiencies in a restricted diet, and to compensate for deficiencies incurred in the kind of poor nutrition which initially led to the weight gain.

There is a third purpose, which requires some explanation, for it involves an enzyme chemistry which to my knowledge has never been invoked to help weight reduction. It is possible that easy conversion of carbohydrate into fat may be influenced by an inadequate supply of the enzymes in the cytochrome P-450 system. These enzymes, important in detoxifying noxious chemicals in the body environment, aren't present in identical quantities in human beings or, for that matter, in animals. That's one reason why we show so many individual differences in our abilities to tolerate chemicals and drugs. It's also a possible reason for a lifetime of steadily increasing difficulty in avoiding or reversing weight gain. Animals deficient in the cytochrome P-450 system will become markedly obese on diets which don't have that effect on animals well supplied with those enzymes. Moreover, as they grow older, these deficient animals suffer a continued, slow drop in the enzyme activities, so that the tendency to obesity becomes stronger as age increases. This is curiously close to the experience of many overweight people, who will tell you that aging brings greater problems with increasing weight gain and greater difficulty in losing weight. But some unpublished data gave me a possible clue to reactivation of the cytochrome P-450 system by use of supplements of lecithin, choline, and inositol. These are "lipotropic"—fat-moving—nutrients, normal to the body. I have heard of sudden success in weight loss in the obese treated with these nutrients. These were not controlled experiments, but the factor of suggestion could not have been operative because the nutrients weren't given to help reducing. I have also observed that when these factors are used as supplements to a low-carbohydrate diet, they tend to point the reducing effect more accurately at the "problem areas." That is to say, they seem helpful in redistributing body fat toward the normal, and sometimes the effect has been seen even in individuals who didn't lose weight.

If your problem with weight loss is serious, there are two other facets of human chemistry with which you should be familiar. One of these is thyroid function. An underactive thyroid, the saying goes, is the excuse for overweight caused by too much refrigerator raiding, but the fact is that there are more thyroid problems than the textbooks admit. In Appendix C, under "Disorders of Women," you will find a discussion of a home test for thyroid activity. If you've had a continued problem with easy weight gain and difficult weight loss, the home test is worth exploring.

Finally, there is the chorionic hormone (HCG) approach to weight reduction. A famous specialist long ago realized that a hormone, the chorionic gonadotrophic, produced in enormous amounts in pregnancy, has the ability to draw fat out of the fat cells and nudge it into the metabolic fire. He saw that hormone as vital to the unborn, who "feed" constantly, although the mother's stomach may on occasion be empty, and who must therefore be able to draw upon the maternal fat reserves to sustain the phenomenal prenatal rate of growth. The physician applied that principle to very stubborn cases of obesity, including those where fat accumulates in tremendous amounts in some areas of the body but not necessarily in others. His method involves a few days of carbohydrate stuffing as a prologue to eating a diet of only 500 calories daily, supplemented with injections of the chorionic gonadotrophic hormone, the doses being a fraction of the pregnancy levels of the factor. In its usual obstructionist way, the American Medical Association condemned the procedure on the grounds that *anyone* will lose weight on 500 calories daily. This is true, but they will also be ravenously hungry; yet with the chorionic hormone treatment, there is no hunger, for the good reason that the patient's actual calorie needs, beyond the 500 from the diet, are supplied by burning his own fat. There are some physicians who have not yielded to peer pressure and give the treatment in appropriate cases. They are often successful, which is as might be expected, for when a member of my medical staff visited the reducing specialist in Rome, he was treating his millionth patient! One does not build a practice of such dimensions on ineffective treatment. There is no listing, unfortunately, of the medical men who employ chorionic gonadotrophic hormone therapy for obesity. One would have to obtain listings of medical nutritionists, and query individual physicians in such practices.

This discussion has, I hope, helped those of you who have learned by experience that the calorie equation isn't always the inflexible law of reducing. And now for the two diets referred to in this chapter. The first, described in the next chapter, is a standard, well-balanced reducing diet, intended for the person who needs only a modest restriction of calories to lose weight. While it is outlined in terms of three meals daily, those for whom appetite is a problem can save foods from specified meals and use them as snacks between meals. If the food craving is formidable, there are two other aids which the nutritionist uses. One is bran tablets, which help weight loss in two ways: by increasing your sense of satiety, and by accelerating weight loss by a mechanism not yet understood. The bran supplement also, of course, helps elimination, which may be important to those who develop constipation when they reduce gross food intake. Another aid is protein tablets or powders. A small amount of protein, five grams or so, between meals, by helping to keep the body supplied with normal amounts of blood glucose, will help to resist both appetite and fatigue.

For those who are unable to lose weight on the standard diet, the low-carbohydrate diet is outlined in chapter 11. Vitamin and mineral supplements to be used with both diets are covered in chapter 12.

10

The Conventional Low-Calorie Reducing Diet

This diet will safely reduce a normal person at a rate of not over two pounds each week. It is a system of constructive reduction which creates no deficiency, save in calories. The diet is balanced in protein intake, and contains enough fat and carbohydrate to keep body function unimpaired. By the code system employed and the lists of foods, the need for set menus is eliminated and there is no need for counting calories.

Every effort has been made to keep vitamin-mineral intake as high as possible. However, a diet below 2,400 calories is very likely to be deficient in vitamins and minerals—a risk inherent in reducing the gross intake of food. It is recommended therefore that this diet be supplemented. This will not interfere with weight reduction but will help to avoid deficiencies of the type which have made reduction hazardous in the past.

A good way to die young is to reduce too quickly. On this diet, which permits much more generous meals than most, a normal person should lose about 6 pounds a month. On it, some of the author's readers and radio listeners have lost as much as 150 pounds—safely, sanely, and without discomfort.

Breakfast

1 serving of fruit
1 egg or egg substitute
½ slice (thin) whole-wheat toast with ½ level tsp. butter
or

1 glass of skimmed milk
1 cup of coffee or tea (optional; no sugar, cream, or milk)

Eggs and Egg Substitutes

Prepare your egg in one of the following ways:
    Plain omelet
    Poached
    Soft-boiled
    Hard-boiled
    Raw
Substitutes for 1 egg:
    Cottage cheese (4 Tbs.)
    Lamb chop (1 small, lean)
    Lamb kidney (1)
    Calf's liver (2 oz.)
    Mutton chop (1 small, lean)
    Buttermilk (1 glass)
    Skimmed milk (1 glass)

Lunch

1 helping of lean meat, fish, fowl, or meat substitute
1 vegetable from Vegetable List A
1 salad (from salad list)
1 serving of fruit or dessert
1 glass of skimmed milk or buttermilk
1 cup of coffee or tea (optional; no sugar, cream, or milk)

Meat Substitutes

Cottage cheese (2/3 cup)
Eggs—poached or omelet (2 eggs)
Buttermilk (2 cups)
Whole milk (1 cup)
Skimmed milk (2 cups)

Dinner

1 cup of soup (optional)
1 helping of lean meat, fish, fowl, or meat substitute
2 vegetables from Vegetable List A plus 1 from Vegetable List B

or

1 vegetable from Vegetable List A plus 1 from Vegetable List B

plus

1 helping of salad (Salad List)
1 portion of fruit or dessert
   Coffee or tea (no sugar, cream, or milk)

Soup List

Consommé
Clear vegetable soup
Beef broth
Chicken, mutton broth
Other clear soups

Note: No creamed soups, none with milk or containing vegetables, meat, or cereals

Fruit List

Orange (small)
Grapefruit (½ medium)
Apple (1 small)
Pineapple (2 average slices)
Peach (1)
Cantaloupe (½ medium)
Melons (2-in. section of average-size melon)
Tangerines (1 large)
Berries (½ cup)
Apricots (2 medium)
Grapes (12)
Cherries (10)
Pear (1 medium)
Plums (2)
Nectarines (3)
Persimmon (½ small)

Fruit Juices:
Grapefruit, Orange (unsweetened;
  6 oz. or 3/4 of water glass)

Vegetable List A

Asparagus (fresh or canned; 8)
Stringbeans (½ cup)
Wax beans (½ cup)
Beet greens (2 heaping Tbs.)
Broccoli (1 5-in. stalk)
Brussels sprouts (½ cup)
Cabbage, cooked (½ cup)
Cabbage, raw (¾ cup, shredded)
Cauliflower (½ cup)
Celery (5 stalks)
Chard (½ cup)

Chicory (½ cup)
Eggplant (½ cup)
Endive (10 medium stalks)
Green pepper (1 medium)
Kohlrabi (2 heaping Tbs.)
Leeks, chopped (⅓ cup)
Lettuce (10 leaves)
Radishes (5 medium)
Sauerkraut (½ cup)
Spinach (½ cup)
Tomatoes, fresh (1)
Tomatoes, canned (½ cup)
Tomato juice (4 oz.; ½ cup)
Watercress (10 pieces)

Vegetable List B

Beets (2 heaping Tbs.)
Carrots (2 heaping Tbs.)
Chives (6)
Dandelion greens (3 heaping Tbs.)
Kale (2 heaping Tbs.)
Onion (1, small size)
Parsnips (2 heaping Tbs.)
Peas (2 heaping Tbs.)
Pumpkin (3 heaping Tbs.)
Rutabaga (2 heaping Tbs.)
Squash (2 heaping Tbs.)
Turnips (2 heaping Tbs.)

Meat List

Lean beefsteak (¼ lb., about 1-in. thick, 2½-in. square)
Roast beef (2 slices, about 3-in. square, ¼-in. thick)
Beef liver (1 slice, 3-in. square, ½-in. thick)

Beef tongue (2 average slices)
Beef kidney (¼ lb.)
Hamburger (¼ lb.)
Calf's liver (¼ lb.)
Lamb kidney (2, average size)
Lamb chop (1, about 2-in. square, ½-in. thick)
Roast lamb (1 slice, 3½-in. square, ¼-in. thick)
Mutton chop (2, medium size)
Boiled mutton (1 slice, 4-in. square, ½-in. thick)
Roast veal (1 slice, 3 in. by 2 in., ¼-in. thick)
Veal cutlet (1, average size)
Veal kidney (2, average size)
Chicken, white meat (2 slices, 4-in. square, cut very thin)
Chicken, broiler (½ medium size)
Chicken gizzards (2, average size)
Chicken livers (2 whole, medium size)

Fish List

Sea bass (¼ lb.)
Bluefish (¼ lb.)
Cod, fresh or salt (¼ lb. to ½ lb.)
Flounder (¼ lb. to ½ lb.)
Haddock (¼ lb. to ½ lb.)
Halibut (¼ lb.)
Kingfish (¼ lb.)
Pike (¼ lb.)
Porgy (¼ lb.)
Red snapper (¼ lb.)
Scallops (⅔ cup, raw measurement)
Shrimp (⅔ cup)
Smelt (¼ lb.)
Weakfish (¼ lb.)
Clams, round (10 to 12)
Crab meat (1 crab or ¾ cup flakes)
Lobster (½ small lobster or 1 cup flakes)

Mussels (4 large or 8 small)
Oysters (12 large)

Salads

Tossed greens
Watercress, lettuce, tomato
Radish and watercress
Chef's salad
Pimento and greens
Baked stuffed tomato, with cottage cheese and chopped celery

If butter is omitted from vegetables at lunch, 1 or 2 teaspoonfuls of salad dressing may be used. Divide dressing between lunch and dinner salads. Two daily are a good idea, for they increase your feeling of satiety.

Desserts

Other than low-carbohydrate fruits such as strawberries and most of the melons, there is no such thing as a low-calorie dessert which a nutritionist with a conscience can recommend. (I'm not about to feed you on gelatin, colored with coal-tar dyes, artificially flavored and sweetened.) Whole gelatin, with added low-carbohydrate fruits, may occasionally be used. If you wish to chance occasional use of saccharin, you will find that low-calorie gingerale added to nonfat milk powder will help slake the sweet tooth. But if you must use artificially sweetened desserts and drinks, do it with discretion, for abuse of saccharin, in the light of all the evidence, is gambling, particularly for men. If temptation is the only thing you can't resist, some of the following devices for controlling appetite should help you.

Hunger Halters

There are nutritional techniques to cope with the yen for sweets, and there are effective behavior modifiers which help to keep you from overeating. In the health food stores, you will find unsweetened protein powders and tablets. You will note that I did *not* mention the protein liquids. The omission is thoughtful. Many (I think virtually all) of these are "collagen"—which is a fancy disguise for gelatin. Gelatin is not a complete protein and doesn't really slake appetite. (If it did, the French Revolution might have been averted, for they tried to satisfy the starving public with gelatin and necessarily failed.)

The protein concentrates are sometimes "sweetened" with vanilla flavor. This does give the illusion of sweetness, if you must have that. A small amount of the powder in water or, better yet, the *chewing* of a few protein tablets between meals will do double duty in controlling appetite, for it satisfies the urge to snack on something and tends to keep the blood sugar from sagging— which is the trigger for appetite in many people.

Another nutritional aid is bran. Five hundred mg. of bran in a tablet—again, chewed—yields a surprising satiety effect and adds the dividend of avoiding the constipation which sometimes occurs when food intake is sharply reduced. See "Diet Versus Constipation" in appendix C for explicit instructions on using bran. For other supplements see chapter 12.

A technique of major benefit to dieters is behavior modification. Certain characteristics of overeaters make reduction of food intake difficult for them. They don't chew enough; they gulp; they don't really taste food; they tend to read or watch TV or listen to radio when they eat. Chew thoroughly and slowly. Direct your attention to what you're doing, which means bypassing TV and other diversions while eating. Count ten before you move your fork from plate to mouth, and chew each mouthful ten times. Really concentrate on tasting what you're eating. As simple as these measures are, they help.

Finally, *don't* use the appetite-depressant drugs. I don't want to write a whole chapter, which would be required, to give you all the reasons for this piece of advice, and will confine myself to the note that a good part of the action of these dangerous medications comes from their depressing effect on the sense of smell. (When your sense of smell is acute, you're more inclined to overeat.) If you must interfere with that, use an inhaler containing one of the amphetamine-type drugs. There is no point in upsetting the whole body when your target is your nose alone.

11

The Low-Carbohydrate Diet

Lesson #1: a low carbohydrate diet is a real economic threat to bakers of bread and processors of sugar, cereals, and grains. When you read hysterical descriptions of such diets as being radical or dangerous, be sure to ascertain the credentials of the critics. You'll find many of them associated, directly or indirectly, with manufacturers of high-carbohydrate foods ranging from cornflakes to soda pop and candy. A conventional 1,200-calorie reducing diet contains 150 grams of carbohydrate. A low-carbohydrate diet contains about 60 grams. That difference doesn't license hysteria.

Lesson #2: Your first step is to provide yourself with a handbook listing the carbohydrate values of foods. I've published one and there are many others available, most of them in inexpensive paperback form. You need this for the break-in period when you are learning to hold your carbohydrate intake down. I know you think you're familiar with the foods high in starch or sugar, but believe me that there are hidden traps in today's marketplace. Few would suspect the high sugar content of ketchup or the presence of sugar in canned green peas or the fact that Shake 'n Bake is about 50 percent sugar. Most people are astonished to learn that the nondairy "creamers" are 65 percent sugar, and that there is sugar added to some brands of salt. Take nothing for granted, for what you miss will surface on your hips. Get the handbook.

Lesson #3: Count your carbohydrate grams before each meal. Your objective is to stay within range of 60 grams of carbohydrate a day. That isn't as easy as it sounds, until you begin to learn, and can select foods "by reflex." Early you will discover that a glass of pineapple juice represents nearly half your carbohydrate allowance for the day, and to select melon or strawberries in lieu of pineapple and other fruits which are astonishingly high in sugar. You will learn to eat open-faced sandwiches, thereby avoiding one slice of bread, and doubling up on the protein— the cheese, meat, fish, fowl, or whatever constitutes the "filling" of the sandwich. And "filling" is a well-chosen word, for adequate protein intake, rarely provided by ordinary sandwiches, does "stick to the ribs." (Would you accept the ham in a ham sandwich as a portion, say for lunch, if it were served without bread?) You will learn to reach for a bit of cheese instead of a cookie, and you will drop breakfast cereals in favor of protein foods at breakfast.

The 60-gram figure isn't critical; it's a starting point, and reflects my conservative approach. Some people thrive on less; some grow weak and irritable when intake goes down to 20 or 40 grams, and some require more than 60.

The diet specifies 5 teaspoons of vegetable oil daily. Some people take it like medicine, by the spoonful, and some try to use capsules, though that will call for an inordinate number of doses. Most find the vegetable oil enjoyable in its normal habitat—on salads. This intake is a *must*, for reasons I've already explained. Don't use the oil for frying. While there's nothing wrong with properly fried food as such, the heat may change the oil chemically, depriving you of the property for which it is being recommended: that of expediting weight loss and directing the loss toward the problem areas.

This diet is for healthy people. It isn't intended for those whose physicians have ordered low-fat menus. It is divided into six meals for the good reason that this helps weight loss and weight control, and aids in normalizing the body's handling of both sugar and fats. It is also a formidable help for those who can resist anything but temptation, for there is little incentive to cheat when you are never far away in time from a snack or a meal.

When first I experimented with the low-carbohydrate diet about fifteen years ago, I specified margarine as a spread since it's made from vegetable oil. However, my good friend Dr. Richard Passwater has pointed out that there is an abnormal concentration of an abnormal type of fat in modern margarine which actually harms rather than protects the arteries. If you elect to use margarine, I'd prefer that you confine yourself to 1 teaspoonful daily, using vegetable oil to make up the rest of the 5-teaspoon quota. When you buy vegetable oil, be sure it is free of BHA, BHT and other additives. While there is no essential difference in supermarket versus health-food-store oils (they are all overprocessed), those in the health food stores usually are additive-free.

The typical low-carbohydrate menu which follows can be adapted to your own habits, so long as you stay within its limitations. This is to say that you can substitute any protein for any protein, but you can't replace a protein with a fat or sugar or starch. You can substitute one vegetable oil for another, and you can substitute one starch for another. (This doesn't contradict what I wrote before about different physiological effects of the same amounts of different starches. Those differences are in *your* chemistry more than in the foods.) You can't use sugar as a substitute for starch, and that includes any type of sugar. There is no form of that much abused food which isn't dangerous in high dosage, and that includes white, yellow, brown, raw, and turbinado sugars, as well as honey, fructose, molasses, and maple syrup. Sugar is sugar.

In adapting the menu to your own life-style, keep in mind that limitation of gross carbohydrate intake is the active principle in this diet. Ten grams more or less of carbohydrate daily will not prove crucial, but greater deviations from the 60-gram level may be significant, speeding weight loss if lower and retarding it if higher. Your subjective feeling of well-being may vary with such changes. How you feel and the verdict on your scale will be the ultimate arbiters of the correctness of the diet for you.

Consistency in using the diet is crucial. Consistency in weight loss *isn't* crucial. Weigh yourself once a week, lest daily fluctuations unnecessarily plunge you into euphoria or depression.

Sample Low-Carbohydrate Menu

Breakfast

Small orange or half grapefruit
Poached egg with sausages (2; no BHT, BHA, or other preservatives)
½ slice of whole-wheat or other whole-grain bread, with ½ tsp. of margarine or, if preferred, 1 level tsp. mayonnaise
Beverage of choice—coffe, decaffeinated coffee, herb or regular tea. Cream if desired; no sugar

Morning Snack

1 cup skimmed milk
¼ cup creamed cottage cheese If bran is being used, 1 tsp. coarse bran may be stirred into cheese.

Lunch

Clear soup (optional)
Chicken or tunafish salad. Use 4 oz. protein food, 1 tsp. mayonnaise, romaine or bibb lettuce, chicory or escarole (unlimited amounts), plus chopped celery, chopped scallion, sliced tomato.
Any vegetable from approved list.
Brown rice crackers (Obtainable in health food stores; 5 are equivalent to 1 slice bread) If you did not use margarine at breakfast, ½ tsp. can be used. In lieu of this, any nut butter can

be used, ½ tsp. Don't overdo—nuts are high in protein and polyunsaturated fat, but contain considerable carbohydrate.
Beverage of choice

Afternoon Booster

½ cup plain yogurt. If not using bran tablets, coarse bran may be stirred in.
Cheese, natural, not processed, not cheese spread, 1 oz. on 1 small whole-wheat cracker

Dinner

Clear soup (optional)
4 oz. tomato juice
Steak or chops or hamburger or fish (¼ lb. cooked weight)
Approved vegetable
Tossed salad, vinegar and oil dressing.
Strawberries, with Half & Half if desired
Beverage of choice

Evening Snack

½ cup skimmed milk or plain yogurt (bran addition optional in yogurt)
1 oz. any leftover chicken, cheese, meat, fish, or 1 tsp. peanut or other nut butter on 2 brown rice crackers.

Your vegetables will be selected from the following list. Eat a daily minimum of 2 cups, total up to a maximum of 4 cups.

Approved Vegetables

Vegetables marked with an asterisk are good sources of Vitamin C, often rich in other nutritional values, and should be emphasized if they please your palate. Of course, the vitamins in your multiple vitamin supplement will protect you even if you're determined not to eat anything that's good for you.

Asparagus
Avocado
*Beet greens
*Broccoli
Brussels sprouts
Cabbage
Celery
*Chard
Chicory
*Collards
Cucumbers
*Dandelion
Eggplant
Endive
Escarole
Green pepper
Green or wax beans
*Kale
Kohlrabi
Leeks
Lettuce
Mushrooms
*Mustard
Radishes
Sauerkraut
*Spinach
String beans
Summer squash
Tomatoes
Tomato juice
*Turnip greens
Watercress

Approved Fruits

Take two servings of fruit daily, in amounts listed. Those marked with an asterisk are good sources of Vitamin C. Fresh, canned, cooked, or frozen fruits may be used, if they're free of added sugar—artificially sweetened fruit is okay, though. Don't peel fresh fruit—peels are fiber sources.

Apple (small)
Applesauce (½ cup)
Apricots, fresh (2 medium)
Apricots, dried (4 halves)
Banana (½ small)
Blackberries (1 cup)
Blueberries (⅔ cup)
*Cantaloupe (¼ of 6-in. melon)

Cherries (10 large)
Cranberries (1 cup)
Dates (2)
Figs, fresh (2 large)
Figs, dried (1 small)
*Grapefruit (½ small)
*Grapefruit juice (½ cup)
Grapes (12 large)
Grape juice (¼ cup)
Honeydew melon (⅛ medium)
Mango (1 small)
Nectarine (1 medium)
*Orange (1 small)
*Orange juice (½ cup)
Papaya (⅓ medium)
Peach (1 medium)
Pear (1 small)
Persimmon (½ small)
Pineapple (½ cup)
Pineapple juice (⅓ cup)
Plums (2 medium)
Prunes (2 medium)
Raspberries (1 cup)
Rhubarb (1 cup)
*Strawberries (1 cup)
Tangerine (1 cup)
Watermelon (1 cup)

All fruits and vegetables, whether served uncooked or cooked, peeled or unpeeled, should be thoroughly washed before consumption. Pesticide residues help no one and can be reduced significantly by washing.

Protein substitutions may be made as follows. A quarter of a cup of creamed or uncreamed cottage cheese, farmer cheese, or pot cheese may be substituted for 1 ounce of meat. Approximately 2 ounces of meat, raw weight, may be replaced with 1 egg. An ounce of cheddar or other American-type cheese, or the equivalent in other types, can replace about 2 ounces of meat, raw weight. Peanut butter is a good source of protein, but it is also a good source of carbohydrate, and the commercial varieties contain saturated fat. Even if it's one of your favorite snack foods, eat no more than one tablespoon of peanut butter weekly.

12

Supplements to Reducing Diets

Multiple-vitamin–mineral supplements, frequently combined in the same capsule or tablet, are widely available from many manufacturers. The health food store will usually carry a larger variety than other sources. Megavitamin potencies are not necessary, for our objective is to protect you against deficiency. With such supplements, it is desirable to use an additional Vitamin B Complex concentrate. Desiccated liver is a good choice. The carbohydrate content of brewer's yeast makes this ordinarily excellent supplement, undesirable with a low-carbohydrate or restricted-calorie diet. A Vitamin B Complex capsule or tablet will be a helpful addition. While some of its values overlap those of the multiple supplements, there are vitamins which frequently are supplied in larger amounts than in the multiples, and some which occasionally are not provided at all in the so-called all-inclusive formula.

The inositol and choline potencies supplied by the multiple and B Complex supplements should be totaled. If they fall short of 500 mg. of inositol and 1,000 mg. of choline in the daily intake, add enough of the vitamins to achieve those levels. Inositol and choline are available in tablets and capsules, individually or combined. Another way to raise choline and inositol levels is via the use of lecithin granules or capsules, which offer the advantage that the choline in this form is less likely to be degraded (broken down) by the bacteria of the bowel. The label on the lecithin capsules or granules should give you the inositol-choline potencies.

Bran is more effective in the coarse rather than the finely ground form. Either form may be obtained in tablets as well as "loose." A detailed description of the way in which to introduce bran will be found in Appendix C. Please note that in reducing diets bran is used not for only its laxative effect but for its favorable effect on satiety (appetite-suppressing) and weight loss.

The odds are long that in the preceding pages you should have found your solution to your weight problem, whether in the conventional reducing diet, the low-carbohydrate menus, stimulation of the enzyme systems, rectification of a thyroid problem, or the use of the chorionic gonadotrophic hormone. May I suggest that I hope to see less of you?

Appendix A:
Notes for the Professor's Letter

The Professor's Symptoms

Episodes of the following in various combinations, almost always occurring between 10 A.M. and 1 P.M., beginning roughly one or two hours after breakfast: extreme anxiety, tightness and pain in chest, shortness of breath, tremor of limbs and internally, fast pulse (some irregularity), cold and sweating hands, pain in stomach, dizziness, nausea, headache, ringing and humming in ears, and fatigue. On a number of occasions these symptoms had become severe, resulting in rhythmic seizures involving violent shaking, rigidity of limbs, coldness, gasping, and total panic, culminating in unconsciousness after injections of Valium.

Sources Referred to in the Letter*

Alexander, F., and Portis, S. A. "A Psychosomatic Study of Hypoglycemia Fatigue." *Psychosom. Med.* 6:191–205, 1944.

*The bibliography accompanying the professor's letter, for the benefit of readers who must verify the incredible for themselves, is far from complete. It does not include, for instance, tests of thousands of "healthy" young men which showed a 14 percent incidence of hypoglycemia, which, of course, was simply explained away by the medical establishment as indicating that low blood sugar is so common it must be *normal*.

Anthony, D., Dippe, S., Hofeldt, F. D., Davis, J. W., and Forsham, P. H. "Personality Disorder and Reactive Hypoglycemia, a Quantitative Study." *Diabetes* 22: 664–675, 1973.

Conn, J. W. "Functional Hyperinsulinism. A Common and Well-Defined Clinical Entity Amenable to Medical Management." *J. Michigan Med. Soc.* 46:451, 1947.

————, "Interpretation of the Glucose Tolerance Test. The Necessity of a Standard Preparatory Diet." *Am. J. M. Sc.* 199:555, 1940.

————, and Seltzer, H. S. "Spontaneous Hypoglycemia." *Am. J. Med.* 19:460–78, 1955.

"A Discussion of Dizziness," The Los Angeles Foundation of Otology (no bibliographical data).

Donnelly, G. L., and Palmer, Y. S. "Functional Hypoglycemia." *South. Med. and Surg.* 106:363, 391, 1944.

Fabrykant, M. "The Problem of Functional Hyperinsulinism or Functional Hypoglycemia Attributed to Nervous Causes," 1. "Laboratory and Clinical Correlations." *Metabolism* 4:469–479, 1955.

————, "The Problem of Functional Hyperinsulinism or Functional Hypoglycemia Attributed to Nervous Causes," 2. "Dietary and Neurogenic Factors, Diagnostic and Therapeutic Suggestions." *Metabolism* 4:480–490, 1955.

Fredericks, C., and Goodman, H. *Low Blood Sugar and You.* New York: Constellational International, 1969.

Gyland, S. Letter, *JAMA*, July 18, 1953.

Harris, S. "Clinical Types of Hyperinsulinism." *Annals of Internal Medicine,* 562–569, 1934.

————, "Hyperinsulinism and Dysinsulinism." *JAMA* 83:729–733, 1924.

Harrison, T. R. *Principles of Internal Medicine.* New York: The Blakiston Div., McGraw-Hill Book Co., 1962.

Hofeldt, F. D., Dippe S., and Forsham, J. W. "Diagnosis and Classification of Reactive Hypoglycemia Based on Hormonal Changes in Response to Oral and Intravenous Glucose Administration." *Am. J. Clin. Nutr.* 25:1193–1201, 1972.

154

Lefebve, P. "Multi-Hormonal Determinations in Hypoglycemia," a lecture delivered at Vanderbilt Hospital, June 18, 1974.

Rennie, T. A. C., and Howard, J. E. "Hypoglycemia and Tension-Depression." *Psychosom. Med.* 4:273–82, 1942.

Appendix B:
A Listing of Competent Practitioners

Reaching practitioners competent in holistic medicine, preventive and therapeutic nutrition, cerebral allergy, orthomolecular psychiatry, chelation, and applied kinesiology is no easy matter. It is frustrating indeed to call an orthodox medical society and be told, as one of my radio listeners was, that *all* physicians are competent nutritionists. Or that chelation is a new, untried treatment (it's at least thirty years old and has been used beneficially for thousands of patients). Or that orthomolecular psychiatry has been "proved" to be a failure—when it has restored thousands upon thousands of hyperactive, autistic, and "emotionally" troubled children to normalcy as well as tens of thousands of schizophrenics and innumerable neurotics, manic-depressives, and other "mentally ill" to effective functioning and good mental health.

For that reason, I am supplying the names of medical and other professional groups whose memberships specialize in these and other areas. When you write to them for a referral, be sure to specify the type of practitioner you wish to consult, and be helpful by enclosing a stamped, self-addressed envelope.

156

Society For Clinical Ecology
Dr. Robert Collier, Secretary
4045 Wadsworth Boulevard
Wheat Ridge, CO 80033
Membership comprises physicians who track down environmental factors which depress health, cause cerebral allergy, or interfere with responses to therapies.

Academy of Orthomolecular Psychiatry
1691 Northern Boulevard
Manhasset, NY 11030
Membership consists of psychiatrists and other professionals who recognize that the body affects the mind. Maintains a list of practitioners, available on inquiry.

International Academy of Preventive Medicine
10409 Town and Country Way
Houston, TX 77024
Membership of health-care professionals, including physicians, dentists, psychiatrists, psychologists, and others interested in holistic medicine, nutrition, preventive medicine, kinesiology, and allergies. Will refer to practitioners on inquiry.

American Academy of Medical Preventics
2811 L Street
Sacramento, CA 95816
This is the society devoted to the study of chelation as a technique of treatment in vascular and cardiac (heart and blood vessel) disorders, such as atherosclerosis. Maintains a referral list.

International College of Applied Nutrition
Box 386
La Habra, CA 90631
Physicians and other health professionals interested in applied nutrition. Will refer.

International Academy of Metabology, Inc.
c/o Kaslow Medical Self-Care Center
2235 Castillo Street
Santa Barbara, CA 93105
  Members concerned with ecology and nutrition.

International Academy of Biological Medicine, Inc.
P.O. Box 31313
Phoenix, AZ 85404
  Health-care practitioners using biological approach in disease
and health. Will refer.

International College of Applied Kinesiology
586 Michigan Bldg.
(Dr. George Goodheart)
Detroit, MI 48226
  Health-care practitioners interested in applied kinesiology.

The Institute of Behavioral Kinesiology
376 F Jeffrey Place
(Dr. John Diamond, M.D.)
Valley Cottage, NY 10989
  Health-care practitioners interested in behavioral kinesiology.

  For those desiring information on environmental impacts on
allergic individuals:

New England Foundation for Allergic and Environmental Diseases
The Alan Mandell Center for Bio-Ecologic Diseases
3 Brush Street
Norwalk, CT 06850
  Conducts research in and distributes literature on clinical
ecology.

The Human Ecology Research Foundation
720 North Michigan Avenue
Chicago, IL 60611
  Distributes literature and helps research in clinical ecology.

For those who wish information on or referral to practitioners in orthomolecular psychiatry and medicine:

The Huxley Institute
1114 First Avenue
New York, NY 10021

Appendix C:
Treatment for Specific Diseases

Acne

Though drug-oriented dermatologists are using antibiotics instead of dietary control of acne, it has long been known
that the skin tends to concentrate sugar more than does the blood.
A sugar-saturated skin, as any diabetic learns, is an invitation to
infection, which is part of the problem (but an important part)
in acne. Sugar also decreases the body's ability to get rid of
bacteria, for the amount of sugar in a king-sized bottle of soda
pop will depress phagocytosis (the ability of the white blood cells
to engulf and destroy bacteria) for hours. This explains why the
low-carbohydrate diet, as free of sugar as possible, has been helpful to some acne sufferers. What carbohydrate is ingested is in
the complex (starch rather than sugar) form. It is also unprocessed, which means using the whole grains—brown rice, whole
wheat, whole barley, whole oats, whole rye, and buckwheat. In
addition to avoiding sugar, it is urgent that acne sufferers be
investigated for sensitivity allergy, or intolerance to foods, which
can aggravate any disease, particularly a skin disorder. A quick
home test for allergy is the pulse-rate method, concerning which

you will find a paperback book by Dr. Arthur F. Coca, *Pulse Test* (New York: Arco Publishing Co., 1968). There are also kinesiological tests for food as well as vitamin and other types of intolerance. These methods are less trying than the conventional scratch-and-patch tests, and may be more accurate, with fewer false positives and fewer false negatives. (See the section on "Allergy" for more information.)

Vitamin A in doses of 10,000 units daily has helped to control acne, but the medical nutritionist may wish to employ more. Despite the propaganda campaign which has so grossly exaggerated the "toxicity" of this vitamin, there are those of us old enough to remember when virtually all infants were given a teaspoonful of cod-liver oil daily. They grew up, although the Vitamin A potency of a high-grade cod-liver oil may reach 30,000 units per teaspoonful. Vitamin A *can* be toxic, of course, but so can anything if overdosed—even water. So don't be astonished if your medical nutritionist takes you up to 100,000 units of Vitamin A daily. He will monitor you for signs of toxicity, for they are reversible when expertly managed.

Zinc, preferably in the chelated form, has been beneficial. Supplementary intake of zinc ranges from 15 mg. to 30 mg. daily, but the physician may increase that. Much higher doses require a compensating rise in the calcium intake, since the two minerals are antagonistic. That antagonism has been used to good advantage when zinc has been employed to remove calcium spurs and deposits.

Vitamin B_6 (pyridoxin) was reported years ago to be helpful in reducing the oiliness of the face, often part of the acne problem. Supplementary amounts of the vitamin range from 5 mg. to 50 mg. daily. The physician may wish to employ more, particularly if the patient shows marked sensitivity to small amounts of sunshine.

Mentioning sunshine reminds one that the summer brings with it improvement of the skin in some cases of acne. This has been responsible for the physician's recommendation of the wintertime use of a sun lamp. Follow the doctor's orders, for excessive exposure yields more penalties than dividends.

161

If the small blood vessels tend to enlarge and become disfiguringly visible, help is sometimes yielded by Vitamin C, up to 250 mg. daily, and citrus bioflavonoids, up to 1 gram (1,000 mg.) daily. These are supplementary doses, and the medical nutritionist may employ multiples of them. Sometimes he will continue to raise the dose until the vitamin causes a laxative effect, after which he returns to the previous dose which did not cause that effect. This, incidentally, is one of the very few "side reactions" attributed to Vitamin C which have a basis in fact. The majority of the others are theoretical products of antivitamin establishment minds. Ask them for case histories to validate their statements, and you will listen to silence.

There *is* a nutrient which can aggravate acne: iodine, or iodides. For that reason, foods rich in iodine and supplements containing it have long been tabooed for these patients. However, recent research indicates that iodine aggravates acne because it interferes with the action of an enzyme of which the vitamin niacinamide is a part. Raising the enzyme level with supplements of niacinamide, therefore, sometimes will offset the undesirable effect of the iodides. One hesitates to deprive the body of this essential mineral because of its importance to the thyroid gland, which is in turn important to the skin. Niacinamide is used in supplementary amounts of 50 mg. daily, but the medical man may wish to raise the intake beyond that level.

Allergies

The time-honored explanations of allergy—antibody-antigen reactions, in the classical lingo—are logical but don't explain all allergic reactions. The time-honored remedies for allergy are largely ineffective, and the traditional tests for allergy were always unreliable. For all these reasons, we're going to bypass the "accepted" approach and explanations and go straight to new methods for identification, relief, and—sometimes—cure of allergies.

Noted elsewhere are two approaches to recognizing the environmental factors that touch off your allergic reactions. These include the pulse-rate method, mentioned under acne, and the kinesiological technique, which relies upon weakening of "indicator muscles" when you are exposed to something to which your body is intolerant. The "muscle method" is so new and startling that not only have many professional and laymen never encountered it, they often refuse to believe what they have seen. But the method *does* work. An oversimplified example of the technique is the arm-strength test. In applying it, you hold one arm parallel with the floor and have someone attempt to press your wrist and arm down. This is not a test of strength but more akin to appraising the resilience of a spring. In the opposite hand, hold the food you are testing—a little sugar, for example—and repeat the "springiness" test of the other arm. If it markedly weakens, sugar is a food to which you are intolerant. When a kinesiologist, who may be a physician or a chiropractor, performs this investigation, he doesn't rest on the reaction of just one muscle system but employs many. The point is that it works, and is frequently more reliable than the conventional scratch-and-patch tests which have long dominated allergy investigation. If you'd like to learn more about it, read Dr. John Diamond's book *BK—Behavioral Kinesiology* (New York: Harper & Row, 1979).

The medical nutritionist also employs other new tests for allergy, one of which demonstrates the adverse effect of allergenic foods or other substances on your blood cells. An alternate method is to put you on a fast and then introduce foods one at a time, thus checking the effects of each addition to the diet. Many physicians dislike this method because it rests on the subjective reactions of the patients—on the symptoms you report, which may be purely internal, after being challenged with a food you don't tolerate. Thus the doctor feels uneasy about the validity of a test when he must ask you if the food gave you a headache, a feeling of nervousness, a tendency to weep, or whatever. The same objections have been raised to sublingual testing, in which a solution of the food, chemical, drug, or vitamin is placed under your tongue, where it is quickly absorbed. Once again, the doctor must rely on your subjective symptoms.

There's nothing really wrong with either of these methods,

since subjective symptoms can be a valuable guide to the effects of the test substance on the body. But medical men like tests which can be objectively appraised. Such a method has now been found, one which invokes a "neutralizing dose," a concept which I must explain before going on to describe the new test. We have learned that a great dilution of the offending substance—much weaker than that used under the tongue—sometimes will cancel all the symptoms of the allergy for many hours. That observation has been combined with the traditional "scratch test" technique of allergists to offer a very accurate diagnosis of allergy and, astonishingly, complete control of the allergic reaction—not just for hours but permanently. In this technique, six injections of the test substance in various dilutions are administered subcutaneously (under the skin). The first three, which are stronger dilutions, reveal the intensity of the allergic reaction, gauged by the size of the weal (hive) that results from the injections. The next three, which are weaker dilutions, usually reveal the "neutralizing dose." When this dose is given by injection rather than by mouth, allergic symptoms are often brought under complete control, not transiently, but permanently.

To illustrate the applications of the "neutralizing dose," let me note first that allergy to food can be addictive: i.e., what you strongly crave may be that to which you are allergic. In that case your craving has two purposes: (1) to get the "lift" an allergenic food gives you, which is why it may accelerate your pulse; and (2) to avoid the withdrawal symptoms, which can make you feel terrible. Let us assume that your allergic addiction is to chocolate, evidenced by the fact that you feel very uncomfortable when you crave it and can't obtain it. If you are given a neutralizing dose of chocolate, which may be as little as a pinhead in a half-glass of water, your craving may totally disappear for many hours. This technique has been used successfully to overcome the alcoholic's craving for whiskey, and is sometimes successful, indicating that the particular patient's problem is allergic addiction to alcohol.

If you'd like to learn more about the effects of allergy on the brain—only recently recognized and long mistaken for neurosis or even psychosis—and more about these newer methods of testing, read *The Food Connection*, (New York: Bobbs-Merrill, 1979), by Drs. Michael Schachter and David Sheinken.

One can understand that new approaches to the ancient problem of allergy will encounter the usual cultural lag in medicine and nutrition, the usual gap in years between a discovery and its acceptance and application. But I do not understand why, for instance, no one has applied nutritional therapies for allergy which were found successful and reported more than twenty years ago. At that time, a researcher named Adams showed that supplements of Vitamin B Complex and predigested protein, both in sensitized animals and in patients with intractable multiple-food allergies, reduced or eliminated completely many of these adverse reactions.

Temporary but gratifying relief from allergic reactions has sometimes been achieved with Vitamin C and Vitamin B_6, taken simultaneously. The doses used by the medical nutritionist may go up to a gram (1,000 mg.) or more of Vitamin C, and as much as a gram of Vitamin B_6. These are, of course, not supplementary but medicinal levels of the nutrients. I have applied the principle preventively, having learned that generous intake of these factors before and after exposure to an allergen—pollen, let us say—minimized or occasionally eliminated the adverse reactions.

Everything I have written in this section will be an exercise in futility if you fail to realize to what an extent allergies may masquerade as other disorders. Many hyperactive children—perhaps 60 percent of them—are targets for allergy to foods, dyes, and additives which worsen their condition. Reading difficulties can be caused by allergy. Schizophrenia is also worsened, allergy being a factor in more than half the cases. Depression not caused by a life situation can sometimes be traced to allergy to anything from food to plastic kitchen tiling or automobile exhaust, to name a few examples. Allergies can make you tired, irritable, unable to concentrate, and headachy, and can worsen symptoms of unrelated disorders. I am saying flatly that there are those who are mislabeled as neurotic or even psychotic, or as hypochondriacs, who are really exhibits of diagnosis by exclusion which failed to exclude two common problems: hypoglycemia and cerebral allergy. And they are interrelated, for low blood sugar can trigger allergy, and allergy can initiate or worsen hypoglycemia.

Chelation—Often an Alternative to Heart Bypass Surgery

The title of this discussion will startle those who have never encountered chelation. It is a method of treating, among other disorders, hardening of the arteries, and my attitude toward it can be quickly appraised when I tell you that I was elected honorary president of the American Academy of Medical Preventics, a society of physicians who practice chelation.

The term comes from the Greek word for crab. A chelating agent is one which reaches, as if with the claws of a crab, for metals and minerals and carries them out of the body. Nature manufactures natural chelating agents—Vitamin C is an example—and there are synthetic chelating agents, of which EDTA (Ethylene-diamine-tetra-acetic acid) is one frequently used by physicians treating hardening of the arteries. This application of a chelator was discovered, as so many medical breakthroughs are, by accident. Many years ago, a physician was treating lead poisoning with EDTA, relying on its ability to carry the toxic metal out of the body. Several of the lead-poisoned patients also had a heart condition—angina—and reported an unexpected dividend from the chelation procedure: their heart pains diminished or disappeared. It was then that the alert physician realized that he had stumbled on a way of treating circulatory problems created by arteries compromised by atherosclerosis, or hardening of the arteries.

The initial lesion in a hardened artery isn't cholesterol, as you've been led to suppose by vegetable oil and margarine manufacturers. It's an abnormal molecule of sugar combined with protein. When the break in the wall occurs, which conceivably could be initiated by deficiency in Vitamin B_6, some of the fats in the blood deposit there. It is at this point that cholesterol deposits begin. The body then attempts to wall off the problem by paving the surface of the deposit with calcium. So long as the calcium "ceiling" is there, the natural recuperative powers of the body are blocked from reaching and removing the cholesterol-fat materials under the calcium. EDTA, as a chelating agent, removes the calcium. If appropriate steps are taken to correct the patient's diet (and life-style), and lecithin and other lipotropic agents like inositol and choline are then administered, a remarkable improvement in circulation can be achieved.

In the early days of chelation therapy some twenty-five years ago, physicians didn't realize that the treatment could be *too* successful. They had to learn that large doses of EDTA given too rapidly would strip so much debris from the artery walls that the kidneys would be unable to cope with so sudden and concentrated a load of "arterial wall garbage." It was then that EDTA gained an undeserved reputation for being nephrotoxic (toxic to the kidneys). This fable is still repeated by the ignorant and by those who, dedicated to resisting all advances in the time-dishonored fashion of medicine, have attempted to discourage the interest of physicians and the public in a nonsurgical, noninvasive method of treating disorders of the blood vessels and the heart. EDTA today is given in much smaller doses and much more slowly. Treatments take four hours, while the EDTA is dripped into the vein, and three treatments weekly for a number of weeks are routine.

Chelation sometimes fails, as all treatments must. Allergy or intolerance to EDTA do occur, though they are extremely rare. Conversely, I have seen this therapy eliminate the need for bypass heart surgery. I have seen it restore victims of severe angina to health, with complete freedom from pain and vastly improved tolerance for exercise. I have watched it save diabetics from the amputations so common in that disorder. I have talked with families of formerly senile patients who regained intellectual function as a result of chelation-improved circulation to the brain.

There are times when bypass surgery is lifesaving. On the other hand, I am aware that the statistics of survival after bypass surgery don't include some of the patients who survive the operation by a few years and then have a fatal attack. The omission in the procedure is an obvious one: if you repair clogged plumbing by inserting new pipes, but don't correct the aberrant chemistry which caused the initial problem, it must recur. That is why the chelating physician insists on necessary changes in life-style, cessation of smoking, intelligent choice of food, and proper use of vitamin, mineral, lecithin, and other supplements. In Appendix B you will find, among other medical societies, the address of the American Academy of Medical Preventics, which is devoted to research in and the practice of chelation. If cost is a factor, you may be cheered to learn that chelation costs but a fraction of the fees for bypass surgery—but of course you must discuss that with the physician of your choice.

Burns and Bedsores

The application of Vitamin E locally in first aid and in treatment for burns has been so completely ignored by the medical world that they haven't even bothered to give it the usual negative comments. This doesn't refer to a Vitamin E ointment, but to the quick application of the contents of a mixed tocopherol capsule. What this does in first aid for a burn you will believe only when you experience the quick relief from pain and the minimizing of blistering. If applied after the blister has formed, the Vitamin E still relieves pain and promotes healing under the blister in a remarkably short time.

For serious burns, the medical nutritionist, taking the necessary steps to avoid infection, will not only apply the vitamin locally but administer it in large doses by mouth. You read earlier about this aspect of the action of topical application of the vitamin in plastic surgery, to make scars less visible and shorten the healing period. Incidentally, I have also seen that effect demonstrated on scars from wounds of less recent origin. However, I have preached the doctrine to plastic surgeons for years without effect, nor have I been able to persuade surgical supply houses to market spray-cans of a sterile preparation of the vitamin. It is difficult to overcome the professional belief that Vitamin E is nothing more than an overrated aphrodisiac.

The same technique has been used to good advantage to help avoid or to help heal and minimize the pain of bedsores. In both burns and bedsores, the medical nutritionist may also use a spray of a 3 percent solution of Vitamin C, and in both conditions a high-protein diet is fed to provide the protein needed for new growth of tissue.

The Common Cold

Colds can be caused by viruses, bacteria, sexual frustration, anger which can't be expressed, allergies, excessive sugar intake, and heaven knows what else. Experiments with preventing or aborting colds, therefore, can't be compared with one another, for you never know whether both groups were treating two different disorders under the same name. That explains some of the differences in the reports you've read about Vitamin C versus the "common cold." Some of the "negative" reports actually weren't negative, and represent the antivitamin establishment at its worst, willing to distort its findings to discourage the public's interest in nutrition.

Leaving aside propaganda and mystical claims, we know that Vitamin C is a potent virus inhibitor and an effective antihistamine. Since allergies, which involve excessive release of histamine, are frequently involved in colds, and viruses certainly are, it is logical that many people have learned that a high intake of the vitamin reduces the frequency, severity, and duration of colds. (As a friend of Dr. Linus Pauling, I'll tell you that his tenacity in battling his critics in part derives from his personal experience with Vitamin C versus colds, for Dr. Pauling suffered from severe colds all through his adult life until he began to use the vitamin.)

People often ask what dose of Vitamin C is needed to break a cold, to which Dr. Robert Cathcart, veteran Vitamin C researcher, has an interesting answer. He says that there are 20-gram colds, 100-gram colds, 50-gram colds—in other words, the dose is determined by the potency of the disturbance. He finds the dose of Vitamin C which causes diarrhea and instructs the patient to stay below that. This may be as much as 50 or 60 grams daily in aborting a cold or as little as 250 mg.

Both from the literature and from personal observation, I have learned that Vitamin A will also break colds. About 200,000 units daily will be required for about five days—too short a period for toxicity to be a concern. There is a twist, however, in this alternate approach, for some people are Vitamin A responders and some are not, just as some are Vitamin C responders and some are not. For sound technical reasons, when one doesn't know his "type," we begin with Vitamin A. If it fails to break that cold, we use Vitamin C for the next cold. The two are not used together, for my experience is that they are antagonists and tend to lower the intensity of the cold but prolong the duration if employed simultaneously.

High doses of Vitamin A for brief periods have also proved helpful for some of the complications of colds such as clogged Eustachian tubes, particularly when this interferes with hearing.

While the Vitamin C enthusiasts recommend the vitamin for bronchitis, this doesn't jibe with my experience. I have particularly noted that an individual who is a Vitamin A responder will, if he switches to Vitamin C to break a cold, bring the infection down into the chest and *cause* a bronchitis. (That's why the individual who doesn't know to which vitamin he may respond should begin with Vitamin A. If he's not the A type, the only penalty will be failure. If you start with Vitamin C and you're an A type, you may wind up with a cough.)

Despite all the space I've devoted to aborting colds, my prime interest remains prevention. Adequate intake of both Vitamin A and Vitamin C will reduce the incidence, severity, and duration of colds. Ten thousand units of Vitamin A daily will constitute a significant protection, the requirement having been estimated as falling between 5,000 and 30,000 units daily. From 250 mg. to 2,500 mg. of Vitamin C daily has been estimated as the optimal requirement.

Colitis, Ulcerative Colitis, Crohn's Disease (Regional Ileitis), and the Irritable Bowel

The notes you are about to read are brief, but they have provided accelerated healing, improved function, given significant relief from pain and distress, and improved response to medication in many individuals with the "melancholy disorders of the bowel" so frequent in the Western world.

Zinc supplementing—15 mg. to 30 mg. daily, or much larger doses as prescribed by the medical nutritionist—has proved to be a source of healing.

Supplements of pantothenic acid—up to 50 mg. daily, or much larger prescribed doses—have restored function in paralysis of the colon.

The use of generous amounts of vacuum-dried or solvent-extracted duodenal (colon) tissue has demonstrated remarkable healing action in colitis and ulcerative colitis. This material tends to be constipating, which is useful when the movements are loose and frequent, but the intake obviously must be gauged to meet the patient's needs. There is no "dose," since colon tissue is food, but amounts needed are usually generous. The tablets are pleasanter to use than the tissue itself, but obviously are less convenient, considering the quantity needed. It might be mentioned that both dried colon tissue and dried stomach tissue have been found helpful in stomach and duodenal ulcer. It is strange that this innocuous type of treatment is largely unknown to the professions, for such preparations of stomach and colon tissues were for years advertised in medical journals. My experience with them is firsthand—I have watched the responses of many patients so treated.

Diet versus Constipation, Diverticular Disease, Appendicitis, Hemorrhoids, and Bowel Cancer

Those who study the incidence of diseases in world populations have been struck by the relative freedom of some primitive groups

171

from such "civilized" and common disorders as appendicitis, varicose veins, constipation, hemorrhoids, diverticulosis, diverticulitis, and bowel cancer. Their immunity appears to be based on diets which provide generous amounts of fiber. There are a number of kinds of fiber in foods, but the type that is most effective is bran (it's noteworthy that you'll find bran in any barn where thoroughbred horses are stabled, for their health is carefully guarded), but bran is missing from the cereals, grains, and flour used by the average family. This triumph of subservience to food technology carries with it a certain ironic overtone, for you must buy the bread, cereals, and flour with the bran removed, and then buy the bran back to cure the constipation you derive from branless foods.

The mischief goes far beyond the constipation caused by a low-fiber diet. Lack of fiber prolongs the journey of food residues to the lower bowel and their exit from the body. In that delay, bowel bacteria are given the opportunity to change certain chemicals in the stool—residues of bile—into unbelievably potent carcinogens (cancer producers). Thus the delicate soft tissues of the colon are for decades bathed in cancer promoters. This, we believe, explains why bowel cancer is so frequent in this country that there are clubs formed by survivors of bowel cancer surgery to induct newcomers into the stresses of the use of an artificial rectum and a colostomy bag.

I'm not interested in constipation alone, although that can be a continuing and torturous problem for some people, but in the threat of the process of which it is an end point. A high-fiber diet, in addition to preventing bowel cancer, may also prevent hemorrhoids, which can be a by-product of straining at stool, as well as diverticulosis and diverticulitis. These are disorders in which, because of such straining, segments of the colon balloon outward. Should those pockets fill with impacted food, the condition can cause great pain.

Paradoxically, for decades a *low*-fiber diet was medically prescribed for diverticulosis and diverticulitis. Now it is realized that such a bland diet may have caused these conditions in the first place, and that apprehension about intolerance to fiber is not justified. About two-thirds of these patients not only are able to tolerate a high-fiber diet, but enjoy dividends of decreased pain. In addition to those in this population who don't tolerate fiber well, there is a percentage of normal individuals—in which I include the constipated as being free from organic disease—who do not tolerate a high-fiber diet. They will necessarily limit their intake of fiber or possibly derive it from fruits and vegetables rather than from the more effective form found in bran. Let me emphasize that these lines, then, are addressed to healthy people, free of organic disease who want to stay that way. If you have hemorrhoids, diverticulosis, or diverticulitis, you are probably under medical supervision and should consult your physician before making changes in diet. If you have nothing more than constipation and you're sure it's no more than that, you're eligible for the plan I am about to present. I call it the BAMBY plan because it includes: *b*ran, *m*ultiple vitamins and minerals, *b*rewer's yeast, and *y*ogurt.

This plan attempts to: (1) change the colon bacteria to a more friendly type, which doesn't attack chemicals in the stool; (2) introduce more fiber and Vitamin B Complex into the diet, since both fiber and these vitamins are important to normal excretion; and (3) provide supplements of multiple vitamins and minerals, useful if one believes that the diet which originally produced constipation was necessarily low in essential minerals and vitamins.

In practice, you begin with the use of bran, in cereal form or tablets. The most effective type of bran is the coarsely ground, whether tableted or not. Two 500-mg tablets are equivalent to one teaspoonful of coarse bran. Intake begins with a single teaspoonful or two tablets after a meal, once daily, and the dose is gradually raised, in tablet or half-teaspoonful at a time, until bowel function becomes *literally* effortless. You may have to raise the intake to three or more teaspoonfuls or six or more tablets daily, in which case it's better to divide the doses among several meals, rather than taking them all at once.

Three warnings: if you show intolerance to bran, such as cramps, stop. Second, in the first two weeks there is a temporary tendency to flatulence (passing gas). This doesn't last, and it must *not* be restrained. You can get into as much trouble with the internal pressures of retained gas as you can with severe constipation. Go to a bathroom, if you must, but vent it. Third, when you become accustomed to bran, don't ever stop it suddenly. Taper off gradually, or you'll encounter the grandfather of all constipation problems for a few days.

Bran may of course be added to cereals or baked into recipes for bread, rolls, muffins, and pancakes. In many recipes, you can substitute bran for 10 percent of the flour. You can also add wheat germ, substituted for up to 2 percent of the flour. Wheat germ is a fine source of B Complex vitamins and of fiber.

Changing bacterial flora in the bowel requires more than the use of yogurt. The quantities needed would be excessive—which doesn't mean that plain (unsweetened, unfruited) yogurt is to be bypassed. Use it, but fortify its action with tablets of the friendly-lactobacillus organisms. Such supplements are available in the health food stores, and the label will specify the recommended intake. Home yogurt makers are also available. It's inexpensive when made at home.

Brewer's yeast, which I employ as a source of Vitamin B Complex, is available in powder and in tablet and capsule form. Be sure that what you buy *is* brewer's yeast and not the *torula* type. If the label doesn't tell you, write to the manufacturer. The distinction is important, for the torula type doesn't supply selenium, which *is* in brewer's yeast. Selenium is regarded as a very effective preventive agent for many types of cancer. So much so that higher levels of human cancer in areas have been found where soil selenium values are low. This correlation occurs 94 times in 100! Brewer's yeast is a food, and there is no "dose," but let me call to your attention the amount fed to severely malnourished (pellagra) patients. It's a quarter of a pound a day. You are therefore not doing something heroic when you take a couple of tablets. Incidentally, some brands of brewer's yeast taste like an accident in search of a victim. Ask the health food store clerk for a palatable brand. You can bake brewer's yeast into recipes too, but don't go overboard—1 percent to 2 percent of the flour content can be discarded in favor of the yeast without materially altering the flavor and texture of the finished recipe. Experiment. It's more fun than a colostomy and much less troublesome. I should mention that brewer's yeast can't be used for leavening.

Multiple vitamins and minerals are, as I noted earlier, available combined in one tablet or capsule, although the dose, particularly if the product is of natural origin, may call for three or more units daily. While there is no chemical distinction between a natural vitamin and its synthetic equivalent, many of the synthetic supplements contain undesirable additives, coal-tar dyes, and sugar, which explains my preference for supplements of natural origin. Then, too, no synthetic concentrate will supply the "co-travelers"—the nutrients which accompany the vitamin in nature. That's one other reason for the use of brewer's yeast.

If you are presently severely constipated, I might be optimistic about the chances of persuading you to adopt the BAMBY plan, or at least of raising your fiber intake. If you're not so troubled, I'm less sanguine but still hopeful. I keep thinking, you see, of the torrent of letters I receive asking if there's any treatment for diverticulitis other than surgery, or any for bowel cancer other than irradiation, chemotherapy, and colostomy. While I can offer some possible help for those who write these letters of desperation, I am driven over and over again to wonder why people aren't motivated by the milligram of prevention rather than the pound of cure. Which is why a recent letter delighted me. My correspondent wrote:

"I am presently in the process of reading your book on high fiber. It's very informative, to say the least. I am a mother of two children and thirty-two years of age. All my life I have suffered from the problem of constipation with no help from doctors who would take this very painful problem seriously. As you said in your book, it's not really paid too much attention by physicians because they don't really consider it detrimental to one's health, only 'uncomfortable' at times. Since reading your book, I find that now I could kick myself for not insisting from my doctor a means such as a high-fiber diet to alleviate this problem.

"All my life I have suffered the interrelated conditions you mention as relating and stemming from constipation as a problem. I have taken laxatives in unbelievable quantities, changed my diet by bombarding it with the fruits and vegetables I could get my hands on, drank prune juice until I sloshed when I walked, until I got to the point of looking forward to my weekly enema. All these results were and still are very discouraging, but the thing that really frightened me was the fact that my younger child has the same problem and up to this point I feared that she would have to be subjected to the same horrors I have been all my life. I sort of became resigned to my situation until reading your book, but having to watch her going through the same pain I could not tolerate.

"There are so many things I endured as a child and adolescent, not to mention an adult, that I now know could have been avoided to a large extent. The appendicitis, the inflamed ovaries, piles, [hemorrhoids], the bleeding at the rectum from stools the consistency of rock, and the list goes on and on.

"After reading only a few chapters of your book I went to a store and purchased a bottle of high-fiber bran tablets, and after taking less than the recommended dose, I have had a bowel movement in less than a day and a half. And better than that—there was none of that awful pain upon evacuation that finally accompanied a movement by other means. I just couldn't believe it. I just had to write to you and tell you that I wholeheartedly support your theory of the value of a high-fiber diet, and hope you will continue your crusade forever. Thank you sincerely, P.A.B."

Diabetes

The treatment of some types of pneumonia might have been much more effective if the search had continued for specific vaccines, but that effort came to a halt with the discovery of penicillin. We could still use the vaccines, for penicillin is far from a panacea in some pneumonias. The case with diabetes is exactly parallel. Had insulin not been discovered, our management of diabetes through other means would have received more study. Yet insulin certainly didn't solve the problem of diabetes, and there are authorities who believe that some of the "complications" of the disorder are actually caused or aggravated by the insulin treatment.

Whether we are discussing juvenile diabetes or the mature-onset type, it has been evident for years that diabetics can benefit by application of modern nutrition. This specifically means repudiating the dogma in diets prescribed by orthodox dietitians and establishment diabetologists. The differences between white bread and whole wheat are patently important for everyone, but critical for a diabetic. The belief that a "well-balanced diet" supplies enough vitamins and minerals is fatuous for those with a high requirement, but can be crippling for a diabetic. The dietitian who makes no effort to persuade a diabetic to choose whole grains is depriving the patient of the help which Vitamin B Complex and fiber—both poorly supplied by white bread—can yield in stablizing blood sugar and reducing insulin requirements. Yet for decades orthodox dietitians have dispensed diabetic diets which list white and whole-wheat bread as equivalents. An error of equal magnitude can be found in the diabetic "food exchange" lists, on which I have already commented, which are based on the proposition that all starches and sugars are identical in their effects on blood glucose and carbohydrate metabolism. This proposition is responsible for diabetics being told that they can interchange starches on the basis of weight: 100 grams of spaghetti for 100 grams, say, of baked potato. The fact is that no two carbohydrates have the same effect on blood-sugar levels, and it is becoming evident that every diabetic should be tested for tolerance to each carbohydrate separately in place of the usual and really outmoded glucose tolerance test.

Recently, the *JAMA* carried an expert's suggestion that a diabetic suffering from a neuropathy, a disturbance of the nervous system common in diabetes, should be given, among other remedies, the Vitamin B Complex. Those aware that what nutrition treats it usually prevents will with justification wonder why all diabetics should not be given the Vitamin B Complex before neuropathies begin. In that group of vitamins, there are factors needed by the nervous system which are essential to the metabolism of carbohydrate, fat, and protein, and at least one vitamin—inositol—which is concerned with the velocity of nerve transmission.

The literature of fifty years ago carried reports on the usefulness of desiccated liver in reducing blood glucose levels. This, like all other therapies, isn't a panacea, but it was found effective enough to encourage the researchers to set up a scale of doses of dried liver as equivalents to given amounts of insulin. The same type of observation was made with choline in the 1940s. I myself, as a consultant to a physician struggling with a difficult case of a juvenile diabetic who had become insulin resistant, watched these therapies reduce the insulin requirement from 160 units a day to sixty, with the lower dose more effective than the higher one in controlling blood glucose levels. Bran has also been found effective in reducing insulin requirements and lowering blood glucose.

The medical nutritionist must often dream of reaching the juvenile diabetic before insulin therapy is started. The opportunity is rare, but it offers the possibility of minimizing insulin dosage. Even if nutritional therapies are delayed until orthodox diet and insulin are started, the medical nutritionist can still help to stabilize a youngster's insulin requirements and to minimize them. He may also perhaps help to minimize if not avoid the "complications of diabetes" to which these children are subject.

In adult-onset diabetes, the nutritionist must often feel exasperated with lost opportunities for prevention. The overweight individual, particularly one with a diabetic history in the family, whose "sweet tooth" is a prominent feature usually needs no medication at all, such as insulin or the oral drugs. These lower blood sugar and present some dangers, like heart attacks, for instance. Reduction to normal body weight, a program of exercise gaited to the individuals needs and tolerance, and the use of desiccated liver, Vitamin B Complex, and Vitamin E will often turn the mature-onset diabetic into a healthier individual. It is important, again, that the B Complex supplement contain more than lip-service amounts of inositol and choline. I stress this not only because these factors are important to liver function, as vital in diabetes as it is in the control of estrogen metabolism, but because many commercial B Complex supplements contain generous amounts of other vitamins but insignificant potencies of these two factors. I recently urged the industry to bring inositol values up to 500 mg. in the daily recommended dose of the supplement, and choline up to 1,000 mg. In response, some manufacturers have done so. Others have introduced tablets containing the two vitamins, sometimes combined with methionine, a protein (amino) acid also important to liver function. Lecithin manufacturers are now emphasizing the fact that lecithin supplies both inositol and choline, and has an advantage in that the bowel bacteria sometimes destroy choline but do not succeed in doing so with the choline contained in lecithin.

Years ago I watched a mature-onset diabetic who refused to stay on a diet and was treated by the means I have just described. Her blood glucose dropped from the 200s to 116, her eyesight improved, and her urine no longer contained "spilled" sugar. She was one of many, but the literature in diabetes continues with its monotonous theme of insulin, oral drugs, and diets which portray white flour as equivalent to whole wheat, white rice as equivalent to brown rice, and vitamin supplements as an option, if that, for the practicing diabetologist to consider. Neglected also is the effect of food allergy in raising or lowering blood sugar, thereby affecting the need for insulin or other drugs.

Gallbladder Syndrome

Of the common disorders of the digestive tract, gallbladder syndrome is probably the greatest source of frustration not only to the patient but to the physician and to the nutritionist as well. The "therapy" has for years consisted of a bland diet free of spices and fiber and very low in fat. Since body functions which are not used tend to atrophy, this "therapy" doesn't improve fat tolerance but impedes it. Ironically, a low-fat diet is an excellent way to develop gallstones, and when they enter the scene, the patient progresses from "functional gallbladder syndrome" to candidacy for surgery. Through the years of this illogically restricted diet, there is often little improvement in the colic, spasm, pain, indigestion, fat tolerance, and constipation. Why would there be? Nor is improvement guaranteed by surgery, however necessary that may be when stones present the risk of chronic inflammation and all the troubles *that* can cause. A survey by a major medical institution showed that nearly 60 percent of all patients who had their gallbladders removed suffered a return of their original symptoms after the operations. To the logician, this might suggest that the trouble was not located in the gallbladder at all.

Certainly this approach, garnished with laxatives and bile salts, is less logical than an effort to improve tolerance to fats and fiber. This is accomplished for some patients by shunning the arbitrary low-fat diet in favor of one which feeds as much fat as the patient will tolerate, with emphasis on vegetable and homogenized fats which appear easier for these people to digest. The focus on the gallbladder alone is discarded in favor of helping liver function, which must be involved when there is poor tolerance to fats. This brings into play the lipotropic factors of the Vitamin B Complex, the familiar Vitamin B_6, choline, inositol, and lecithin which you have encountered so many times in this text. Desiccated liver is also employed as a supplement. Enzymes are used to help utilization of all dietary components, meaning protein, fat, and carbohydrate. These include pancreatin, bromelin, and papain. The net result, and I obviously write from experience, can be a patient free of symptoms, no longer dependent on laxatives and able to eat a normal diet.

Disorders of Women

Before giving you the nutritional guidelines for women, let me restate the objectives. We are bringing estrogenic hormone under the natural control of the body. In so doing, we expect improvement in premenstrual tension and other premenstrual symptoms. We should reduce the length of the menstrual—from five days to three in many women—with a significant reduction in the intensity of hemorrhaging. Transient cysts of the breast—those appearing and disappearing in the weeks from ovulation through the period—may no longer appear, or be reduced in both size and tenderness. Cystic mastitis—more or less permanent cysts of the milk-producing tubules of the breasts—may disappear or be significantly less troublesome. In rare cases, uterine fibroid tumors may become smaller or disappear; in some, growth of the fibroids may halt or be slowed. (This is no more startling than the anticipation of the gynecologist that such tumors may shrink, disappear, or slow in growth at menopause when estrogen activity goes down.) These early dividends from better nutrition are capped by a long-term possibility: the reduction in estrogen activity should lessen significantly the risk of estrogen-dependent cancers of the breast and uterus. Warning: there is no risk in using better nutrition to make the menstrual cycle normal. There *is* risk in treating yourself for disease—cystic mastitis or uterine fibroid tumors, as an example. Neither of us would know, without competent medical supervision for you, whether a cancer may be hiding under the cysts or whether the uterine growths are actually benign. Seek competent medical supervision when using nutrition therapeutically. There are no risks in better diet, but distinct risks in self-diagnosis and self-treatment.

Control of estrogenic hormone is exercised by the liver. You can help to make that process more effective by the following steps:

1. Reduce your intake of all forms of sugar. This includes white, yellow, brown, raw, turbinado, honey, molasses, and fructose. Your present intake, if you're average, is 100 pounds—too much per year.

2. Raise your intake of foods rich in Vitamin B Complex. This means using whole-grain foods in place of white flour, white rice, degerminated corn, processed buckwheat and rye. Select whole wheat, brown rice, whole rye, whole cornmeal, whole

181

oats, and similarly unprocessed grains. At the meat counter, remember that the muscle meat—steaks, chops, and roasts—are low in B Complex vitamins as compared with organ meats, such as liver, kidney, and sweetbreads.

3. Learn to use special-purpose foods rich in Vitamin B Complex and low in calories. These include wheat germ and brewer's yeast. There are secondary reasons for this recommendation. Both foods supply selenium, which is a mineral known to be significantly helpful in resistance to and treatment of cancer. In addition, wheat germ is a rich source of Vitamin E, which also has an anticancer as well as antiaging effect. (Most antiaging nutrients are also protective against cancer.) Be sure the yeast is brewer's. Remember, there is another variety—torula yeast—which does not supply selenium.

4. It is important that your diet supply the protein (amino) acids needed to support liver function. It's a gamble to rely on vegetable sources for these amino acids, which are best and more efficiently supplied by animal protein such as meat, fish, fowl, cheese, milk, and yogurt. Have at least a small amount of such a protein at each meal.

5. Be sure your iodine intake is adequate to protect your thyroid, for hypothyroidism (low thyroid activity) is a risk factor in breast cancer. If you use salt, be sure it's iodized. If you're avoiding or cutting down on salt, as many people do who are concerned about their blood pressure, use kelp tablets or a multiple mineral supplement which includes iodine, usually in the form of an iodide compound.

To check your thyroid function, there's a simple test which can be performed at home. The test is performed on the third day of the menstrual in women in that age bracket and at any time for others. On awakening and before arising, place a fever thermometer (shake the thermometer down the night before) under the arm and keep it here for ten minutes. If the reading for three days in succession is below 97.8° and you have any symptoms of thyroid underactivity, this simple test should direct you to your doctor for appropriate treatment with thyroid hormone.

6. Both for antiaging and anticancer effect, it is desirable to raise the intake of Vitamin E beyond the level obtainable from food. The vitamin should not be used in the alpha tocopherol form usually chosen by the public, for there are three other forms of the vitamin, and all four can be purchased together in capsules called "mixed tocopherols." (The other three forms, beta, gamma, and delta, yield more of the antioxidant effects which are important in the anticancer, antiaging actions we are seeking.) Mixed tocopherols usually carry a potency statement on the label, referring to alpha tocopherol potency. This should be about 200 mg. The amounts of beta, gamma, and delta tocopherols are usually not stated, although they should be.

7. It has already been mentioned that brewer's yeast is a source of selenium. If the yeast is not being used routinely in quantities equivalent to at least one tablespoonful daily, it would be desirable to use a selenium supplement. I prefer "organically bound" selenium rather than such compounds as sodium selenite. The organically bound form usually is described as being derived from brewer's yeast.

8. If you choose to accelerate the process by using a Vitamin B Complex supplement—which is a good idea, since calorie ceilings may prevent you from eating enough of the foods supplying these vitamins—be sure that the supplement, in addition to the usual B vitamins, supplies at least 500 mg. of inositol and 1,000 mg. of choline in the recommended daily dose. If you are already using the Vitamin B Complex and it does not supply these vitamins in adequate amounts, you can purchase inositol and choline tableted together. If you prefer, you can use lecithin as a source of these two vitamins, which I find indispensable in helping the body to control estrogen. This would require an inconvenient number of lecithin capsules daily, but lecithin granules are available, and one tablespoonful daily will be helpful. The granules can be sprinkled on cereal or taken mixed with any beverage such as fruit juice.

9. It will be wise to completely eliminate use of caffeine-containing beverages and foods and those which contain compounds analogous to caffeine. These would include coffee, tea, cola

drinks, and chocolate. There is a chemical—a xanthine—in these products which, for reasons not yet understood, has the capacity to cause breast cysts. Not all women with cysts so caused will have relief by tabooing these drinks and chocolate, but it's certainly worth the try.

10. Not all of women's troubles, obviously, originate with excessive estrogenic hormone activity. Nor will all women who are high-estrogen respond to the high-protein, high Vitamin B Complex regime. Additional steps may be taken by the medical nutritionist to raise the percentage of successes:

a. He may add a supplement of manganese. Supplementary amounts range from 2 mg. to 5 mg. daily, but the physician may wish to employ more. He will watch the patient on higher doses for early signs of tremor, which would reflect intolerance to such levels, and in such cases will reduce the dose.

b. Lack of hydrochloric acid and of protein-digesting enzymes may render the high-protein diet ineffective or less effective than it should be. The nutritionist would meet the need for added hydrochloric acid (production of which in many people, particularly older people, is inadequate) with supplements such as glutamic acid hydrochloride. Enzyme activity will sometimes be raised by appropriate supplements of the enzymes from such sources as pancreatic tablets, papain (from papaya), and bromelin (from pineapple).

c. He may add high doses of Vitamin A.

In the first month of the improvement in diet the body's control system, which is centered in the liver, may not yet have responded as the liver is an organ which lags in response to changes in nutrition. Meanwhile, the output of estrogen, in response to optimal diet, may promptly rise. Thus the first menstrual after the nutrition has been bettered may be *more* disturbed. In the second month, the control mechanism catches up and improvement should begin. When it does, keep in mind what it signifies: estrogen, a cancer-promoting hormone, has been physiologically tethered. I want to reemphasize that this applies to estrogen from any source: the ovaries, the adrenals, the birth-control pill, the estrogen used in the menopause or for menstrual irregularity, that which may be found in traces in animals plied with the hormone to accelerate weight gain, and, finally, estrogen that occurs naturally in food. It may not be obvious, and it should be emphasized that the physician who prescribes estrogen in any form will be helping to protect the patient not only by making it a point to keep the doses at the lowest possible level, but also by using good nutrition to assure proper control of the hormone by the body's regulatory mechanism.

Two final thoughts which must reach you before we close this discussion: (1) The primary responsibility for your well-being does not rest with any government agency, any consumer protection group, or any profession. It is *yours*. (2) You can't fulfil that responsibility unless you resolve to take charge of your own body.

Stop to think: who should really accept the blame when cancer-free breasts are removed in the name of cancer prevention? When a cancer-promoting hormone, estrogen, is prescribed at the rate of $50 million yearly? When attempts are made to persuade mothers to permit mastectomies on newborn babies, or healthy women to undergo castration at age thirty-eight?

P.S. A gynecologist in my home area telephoned as I was writing the preceding lines. He asked for a copy of my text on nutrition in preventing breast and uterine cancer. I asked him flatly why a thoroughly orthodox gynecologist suddenly was showing interest in nutrition for women. His response lends emphasis to everything you have just read. His patient, he said, came to him with what he diagnosed as uterine fibroid tumors. When she received the diagnosis, she told him that she was beginning treatment with a high-inositol-choline B Complex. (There was no need to change her diet, which for years faithfully followed the outline you have just read.) She returned to him recently, and he found to his astonishment that the tumors had disappeared. This was something, he confessed, he had never seen before. Another gynecologist, head of the department at a major New York hospital, had reacted the same way to one of his patients who, as one of my students, proceeded to follow the antifibroid nutrition regime. After five months, he told me, there was no evidence of uterine fibroid tumors. They *had* been there, he emphasized, and they *had* disappeared. "But," he said, "fibroids don't disappear."

Do you remember the story of the child who, seeing a giraffe for the first time, said, "There ain't no such animal"?

Menopause

The National Cancer Institute recently granted that menopausal use of estrogen (female hormone) risks an increase in uterine and, years later, breast cancer. Many physicians consider the risk acceptable on the grounds that estrogen therapy "increases the quality of life" for menopausal women, thereby tacitly granting that the hormone is the *only* answer to the menopausal problems of sweats, flushes, irritability, insomnia, atrophy of vaginal tissues, and weakening of the bones (osteoporosis). Not only, as I have already indicated (chapter 5), is there substantial doubt that estrogen deficiency is responsible for the "hot flashes," but there is evidence that some responses to the hormone are patently a placebo (power of suggestion) reaction. In a well-controlled experiment in which one group of menopausal women were given estrogen and another group "dummy" capsules which the women thought were estrogen, the "dummy" group responded just as well as the hormone group. So not only does female hormone therapy for the menopause rest on equivocal evidence, but it is simply not true that all women are locked into the bleak alternatives of estrogen therapy with its dangers or suffering with sweats, flushes, and decalcification of the bones. In the first place, as you will learn in reading this discussion, there are nutritional safeguards which can be provided for the small group of women who *must* have estrogen therapy, which I should hope would be given in minimal doses. In the second place, there are nutritional and safe medical resources to treat menopausal symptoms, and they usually go untapped. These range from mild sedation—and I count medically supervised administration of barbiturates far less undesirable than estrogen therapy—to supplements of nutrients which include at least one (Vitamin E)

186

which sometimes quiet the hot flashes, often calm the nervous system, restore normal sleep, and prevent, stop, or even reverse postmenopausal weakening of the bones (osteoporosis). In addition to Vitamin E as mixed tocopherols, these include lecithin bioflavonoids, calcium and magnesium orotates, Vitamins A and D, and the Vitamin B Complex as supplements, coupled with the type of good nutrition described in the preceding section.

As I emphasized when recently interviewed by *Harper's Bazaar*, a sensible woman doesn't wait for the menopause to begin emergency nutritional measures. Preparation for it should start no later than the early thirties. A lifetime intake of more than 800 mg. of calcium daily—equivalent to 4/5 quart milk or roughly three ounces of cheese—builds protection against osteoporosis; less than 300 mg. daily invites it. The woman who is poorly nourished, nervous, tense, and anxious as well as the woman with unrecognized or uncontrolled allergies, will have a more stormy menopause than the well-fed woman who has come to terms with life and has recognized the nutritional needs peculiar to women.

Nerve-Muscle Disorders

Anyone who is in any way interested in the healing effects of nutrition must sooner or later be confronted with the long list of myoneuropathies or nerve-muscle disorders. These are widely varied diseases, but they share a characteristic: orthodox medicine has little to offer, and the greater part of what it does provide is symptomatic treatment which, as all such treatments must, ignores cause, never cures, and rarely arrests. Included are cerebral palsy—athetoids, spastics, rigidities, and tremors—as well as multiple sclerosis, amyotrophic lateral sclerosis, strokes, postviral encephalitis, muscular dystrophy, and myasthenia gravis.

Nutritionists have no panaceas and no real cures for these disorders, but food and food factors have yielded very real dividends in some of these diseases, and control of a few. So far, this is an optimistic report on a subject to which I have devoted most of my professional life, for I have specialized in myoneuropathies, driven by the promises of good nutrition and the bankruptcy of the conventional drug therapies. But from this point follows an exercise in frustration. Let me explain.

Many years ago my attention was drawn to the use of a fraction of wheat-germ oil, concentrated for that purpose by the Viobin Corporation at the request of a specialist in muscular dystrophy named Milhorat. For many years, that concentrate of a wheat-germ-oil fraction was known as the Milhorat concentrate. At the time I encountered it, Dr. Ezra Levin, whose research was responsible for isolating and concentrating the factor, informed me that it would probably be useful in other myoneuropathies, but was being used at the time for muscular dystrophy alone. I brought the material to the attention of a group of physicians with whom I was then working, and over a period of years we established its value in the treatment of multiple sclerosis. That in turn, as you have learned from reading the Introduction to this book, led to a trial of the material in cerebral palsy. I then was responsible for application of the therapy by physicians treating stroke victims. Certain observations suggested that this wheat-germ-oil fraction was capable of stimulating the repair of damaged neurones, even in the brain, where such repair is classically described as unachievable. And that brings us to the present. The supply of this fraction has been cut off because the company now finds production too costly. The result has been that many patients here and abroad who have benefited by this harmless nutritional medication have been writing letters of desperation to the distributor. There being no other source of the fraction, which is a long-chain waxy alcohol, I share the frustration of the patients, some of whom owe to this treatment their return to normal activity and now fear becoming invalids again. The problem resolves itself into the arithmetic of the product and the body's tolerance for fat. One could swallow enough wheat-germ oil to yield a therapeutic amount of the waxy alcohol, but few people could tolerate that much fat.

I feel, nonetheless, that you should be acquainted with this history if the subject is of personal importance to you, because it is possible that the concentrated waxy alcohol will be recognized as the valuable therapeutic weapon it is and will shortly reappear on the market. In the interim, we'll have to compromise by using wheat-germ oil, with the stipulation that it *must* be solvent-extracted. The so-called cold-pressed oil doesn't contain enough of the material.

The therapy in multiple sclerosis, then, began with the long-chain waxy alcohol accompanied by Vitamin E and B Complex supplements, with high potencies of choline and inositol. The diet recommended comprised frequent small meals rather than infrequent large ones, with special emphasis on sardines and mackerel. This is not arbitrary; it is based on the fact that the "insulation" shielding the nerves is being stripped away in multiple sclerosis, and a fat found in these fish, preformed, is the first so to be lost. The diet excludes wheat and milk, for many MS patients are intolerant of these foods. While the establishments in multiple sclerosis ignore these findings, they have been applied successfully by many medical nutritionists and embellished with acupuncture, biofeedback, and other helpful techniques in developing which Dr. Arthur Kaslow is probably the pioneer. The important point is that MS patients mustn't surrender to the generally negative approach of the orthodoxy in medicine. We in nutrition *do* get results.

In cerebral palsy, my experience has been confined largely to the spastic type. Control of nutrition and use of nutritional therapies have been productive in improving both neuromuscular and intellectual function, although it should be emphasized that the majority of these children are not mentally retarded. I have found it rewarding to check these children for allergies—particularly cerebral allergies—and to protect them against hypoglycemia. I don't like to give the glucose tolerance test to children, and have persuaded some physicians that one can demonstrate the presence or absence of low blood sugar by therapeutic diagnosis, which means placing the child on the appropriate diet

189

and watching the response. If six weeks brings an improvement in mental or physical performance, one can conclude that hypoglycemia was present and has been controlled. The neuromuscular fraction of wheat-germ oil has produced striking benefits in some of these children. Not only has there been a dividend in better mental and neuromuscular function, but sometimes I have seen muscular strophy (from disuse) reversed. With the wheat-germ-oil fraction, we have used Vitamin E (mixed tocopherols), the Vitamin B Complex (again of the type with high potencies of inositol and choline), and multiple vitamins and minerals as supplements for a high-protein diet low in processed carbohydrates and fed in frequent, small meals. Exactly the same nutritional procedure has been used to help victims of strokes, where the therapy has been augmented by high doses of Vitamin C and bioflavonoids, specifically aimed at strengthening the small blood vessels which frequently, rather than the larger ones, are the target for the "accident" in the brain.

In myasthenia gravis (serious weakening of the muscles), nutrition is employed in a more specific way. The orthodox medical treatment is aimed at increasing the activity in the body of a neurotransmitter, acetylcholine. Some patients don't respond to the drugs which do that; some overrespond and become victims of what is called a "cholinergic crisis." The nutritional method is to increase the acetylcholine activity in the body by providing the precursors from which the neurotransmitter is synthesized there. These are pantothenic acid, choline, and manganese. Unlike the drugs, the administration of the precursors can't cause overproduction of the transmitter and thereby can't cause a "cholinergic" crisis.

Interestingly, the same neurotransmitter is involved in glaucoma, and the pantothenic acid, choline, manganese therapy has been used helpfully in some instances where the miotic drugs (the conventional eye drops) used in this eye disease have lost their effectiveness. High doses of ascorbic acid accompany the glaucoma therapy, since the diuretic (water-excreting) effect of the vitamin may in some individuals also help to reduce the pressure in the eyes.

Some Nutritional "Pearls"

Schizophrenia

Amino acids such as tryptophane offer as much help to some schizophrenics as the vitamin therapies with niacinamide, pyridoxin, and Vitamin E have yielded.

In perhaps half of the schizophrenic population, cerebral allergy and hypoglycemia are present. No schizophrenic can be considered adequately investigated and treated if there has been no check to determine if diet is contributing in any way to the problem.

Lack of hydrochloric acid is present in some schizophrenics. Though this may be relatively an infrequent problem, coping with it has increased the effectiveness of orthomolecular psychiatry in the management of this malignant disease.

The cure rate in schizophrenia is magnificently high with orthomolecular treatment *if* it is started promptly. Delay is prejudicial—long-term schizophrenics are less likely to respond, although some do.

Hypoglycemia

Exercise, such as running on a treadmill, or hyperventilation, by breathing into a paper bag, instituted at the fourth hour of a six-hour glucose tolerance test may elicit symptoms of low blood sugar which otherwise might remain hidden.

When the hypoglycemia diet fails to relieve women of frigidity, the administration of adrenal cortex injections, or the oral equivalent, in the precursor material may prove strikingly effective.

Supplements of glycerin sometimes speed recovery in hypoglycemia.

Avocado contains a type of sugar which not only does not stimulate insulin production but tends to suppress it.

Myopia

Despite orthodox resistance to the concept, eye exercises *do* improve nearsightedness in many myopics. So do large doses of Vitamin D and moderate amounts of calcium, a therapy which should be medically supervised to guard against Vitamin D toxicity.

Gingivitis

While all dentists and most laymen know that Vitamin C deficiency can cause bleeding gums, it is little realized that a Vitamin C deficiency can be caused by an excessive intake of sugar and processed starch, rendering a normally adequate intake of the vitamin insufficient.

Osteoporosis

This subject has been discussed earlier, but I want to add a note of caution which is frequently ignored. When a woman begins to show signs of peridontal disease—loosening of teeth as a result of weakening of the supporting structures, including decalcification of the jawbone—this may be the tip of the iceberg, an early warning that the entire skeleton is being eroded.

Intermittent Claudication

This disorder, common in older people, causes intolerable pain in the legs during brief, mild exercise—even walking. With all the adverse criticism of Vitamin E as the vitamin in search of a disease, the antivitamin establishment has managed to overlook hundreds of papers and clinical observations which clearly show that mixed tocopherols are an effective treatment for the disorder. Moreover, the effects can be objectively measured since the response is in terms of much more tolerance for exercise before pain sets in, and in some cases the pain is eliminated entirely. Fascinatingly, the vitamin is obviously correcting disturbed metabolism in the leg muscles. The heart is a muscle, too, remember?

Vitreous Floaters

This annoying, if usually harmless, disorder creates little specks which float across the field of vision. Orthodox treatment is ineffective. High doses of Vitamin D and calcium—again, necessarily medically supervised—have been reported helpful to some patients. High doses of lipotropes—inositol, choline, methionine—have been reported helpful by another investigator. Discuss these observations with your ophthalmologist.

Index

Acetylcholine, 80
Acne, 160–62
  allergy test and, 160–61
  iodine and, 162
  niacinamide and, 162
  sugar and, 160
  sun lamps and, 161
  vitamin A and, 161
  vitamin B_6 and, 161
  vitamin C and, 161
  zinc and, 161
Alcoholism, 25–26, 83–85
Allergies, 49–50, 162–66
  acne and, 160
  addiction and, 50
  kinesiological test, 163
  "neutralizing dose" test, 164
  pulse-rate test, 160–61, 163
  vitamin B Complex and, 165
  vitamin B_6 and, 165
  vitamin C and, 165
American Academy of Medical Preventics, 166, 168

American Psychiatric Association, 107
Amyotonia congenita, 13
Anatomy of an Illness (Cousins), 121
Anemia, 1
Ankylosing spondylitis, 121
Appendicitis, 171, 172
Arthritis, 3, 15, 112, 114–24
  bee venom therapy, 121–22
  conventional treatment for, 114–15
  eggs and, 122
  niacinamide and, 118
  nightshade plants and, 116–17
  royal jelly and, 120, 123, 124
  supplement dosages, 123–24
  zinc and, 120
Arthritis Foundation, 3, 62, 115, 116, 117, 122
Autistic twins, 107–108

199